Acclaim for

KATHY SMITH'S

flex appeal

"Kathy Smith has gotten right to the heart of the problem
for many women . . . not being connected to their bodies!
This program is a great way to get reacquainted!"

—Dr. Susan Love,
author of *Dr. Susan Love's Menopause & Hormone Book*

"Kathy is a vigilant and inspired teacher, wisely concerned
with both physical and inner well-being. *Flex Appeal* is a tribute
to her knowledge of women and our lives."

—Téa Leoni, actress

"This book is a gem that will change lives for the better.
More than just a book about revving up your sex life, this is a vital
and accessible program that will help you reclaim the life you deserve—
one filled with passion, pleasure, and delight."

—Rod Stryker, yoga master

Also from Kathy Smith and Warner Books

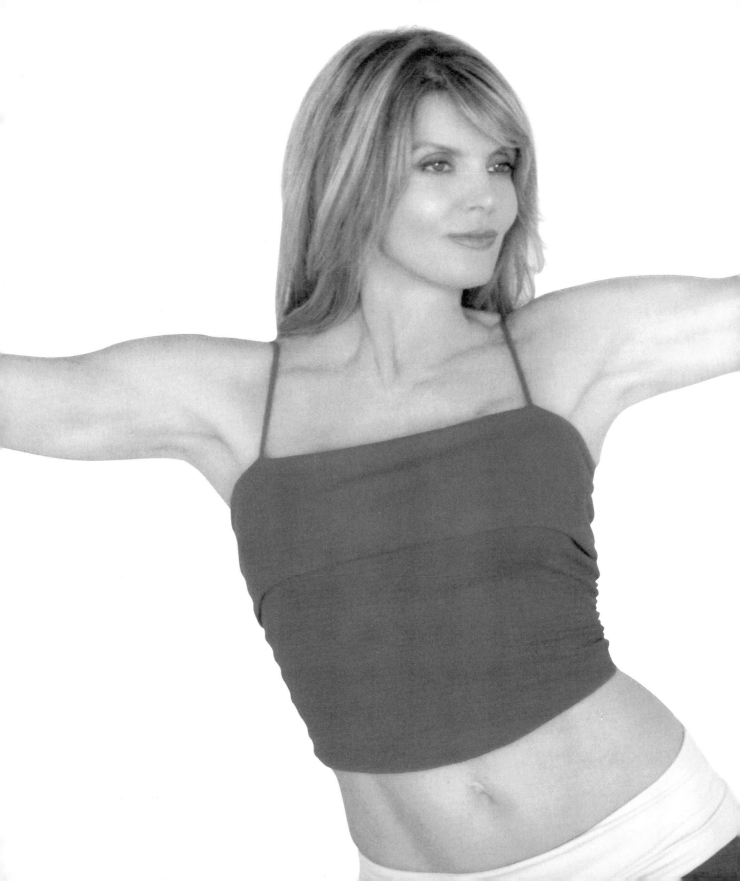

KATHY SMITH'S

flex appeal

LOOK GREAT AND FEEL SEXY AT ANY AGE

Kathy Smith

with Robert Miller

Flex Appeal program created by
Kathy Smith and Micheline Berry

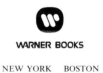

WARNER BOOKS

NEW YORK   BOSTON

Neither this exercise program nor any other exercise program should be followed without first consulting a health care professional. If you have any special conditions requiring attention, you should consult with your health care professional regularly regarding possible modification of the program contained in this book.

Copyright © 2004 by Kathy Smith Enterprises, Inc.
All rights reserved.

Warner Books

Time Warner Book Group
1271 Avenue of the Americas, New York, NY 10020
Visit our Web site at www.twbookmark.com.

Printed in the United States of America
First Printing: February 2004

10   9   8   7   6   5   4   3   2   1

Library of Congress Cataloging-in-Publication Data
   Smith, Kathy.
     Kathy Smith's flex appeal : look great and feel sexy at any age / Kathy Smith.
        p.   cm.
     ISBN 0-446-69228-X
      1. Bodybuilding for women.   2. Exercise for women.   3. Body image.   I. Title:
   Flex appeal.   II. Title
   GV46.6.W64S54   2004
   613.7'1'082—dc22   2003018790

Photography by Cory Sorensen
Additional photography by Antoine Bonsorte
Kathy Smith's wardrobe created by Los Angeles–based designer Elisabetta Rogiani
(www.rogiani.com)
Illustrations and editorial assistance by Amy Zone (www.zoneyoga.com)
Book design and text composition by Ralph Fowler
Cover design by Brigid Pearson
Cover photo Michael Elins

Acknowledgments

To Rob: This is our third collaboration, and each time the process is even more fulfilling. Talking endlessly over cups of green tea and Bay Cities sandwiches, I admire your ability to listen to me, to immerse yourself in the subject matter, and to organize our process. Most of all, you make it fun.

To Micheline: I'm delighted we finally got to work together. I've always respected your expertise in yoga and dance, and I now truly appreciate your magnificent gift. Watching you move is a delight; watching you transform other women's lives is an inspiration.

To Jackie and Matt: Many thanks for your energetic production assistance and for managing all the details that make a project like this run smoothly.

Thanks to Kate and Perrie for supporting me in the process, even though you're not quite sure about the subject matter.

Thanks to all the women who shared their stories during the writing of this book.

Finally, thanks to Diana Baroni of Warner Books, for being open to my stretching into new areas, and for your patience and willingness to stick with the idea through its long evolution to become this book.

Contents

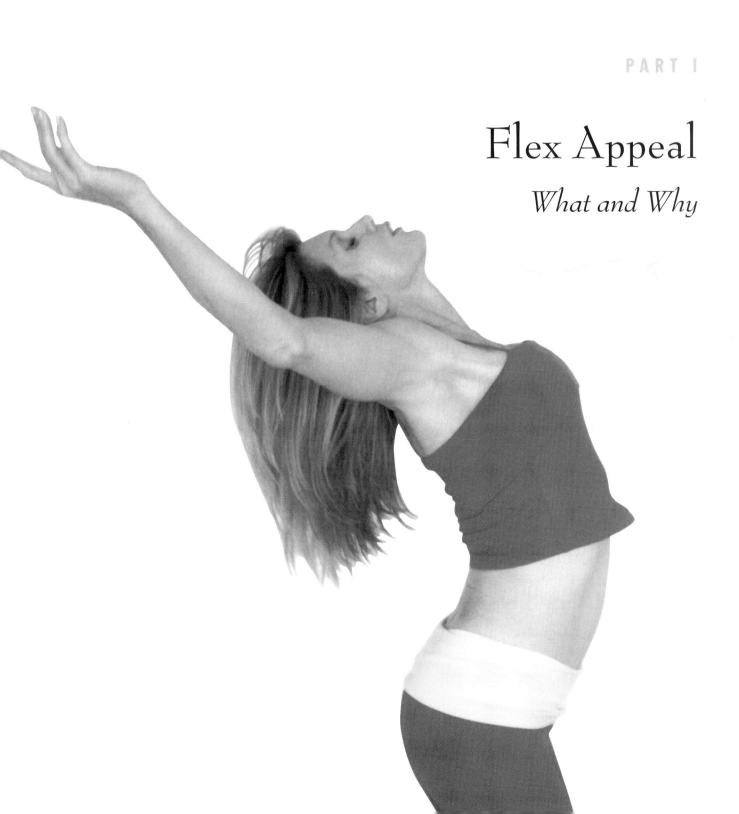

PART I

Flex Appeal

What and Why

CHAPTER 1

My "Opening" Act
The Search for Sensual Vitality

TWO YEARS AGO, having just turned fifty, I set out to write a book about sex. Easier said than done! After exploring the swarm of midlife changes our bodies go through for my book *Moving Through Menopause*, I'd become aware that questions of libido and sexual function are a big concern as we get older. At the same time, I knew of younger women, caught up in the stresses of career or motherhood, who found themselves wondering at the sudden lack of passion in their lives. The truth is, a feeling of disconnection from your sensual vitality can happen at any time, and women of all ages may hear that voice inside them asking: *Is that all there is?*

I knew that much had already been written about these issues, and I was determined to find a new approach.

Promises, Promises . . .

Standing at the magazine rack in my local bookstore, I was struck by our culture's single-minded focus on the mechanics of sex. Every cover screamed *sexual performance*—as though new bedroom breakthroughs were being made every day. *Drive him wild! Make him beg for more!* How could anyone's sex life founder, with so many surefire techniques to try?

But there comes a point when you simply no longer relate to these breathless promises. For someone like me, recently divorced and emerging from a long period of celibacy, the vulnerability and longing associated with the thought of sex were more likely to bring up feelings of anxiety, sadness, or just plain apathy.

Then I was hit by one of those simple-but-brilliant revelations: Before you can really enjoy a sexual relationship, you need to *feel* sensually alive in your own skin. In other words, before you can really be in the mood, you need to be comfortable *in your body.*

Instantly I was on familiar ground, because I saw how this concept dovetailed with my mission in the fitness field: The issue wasn't about *having sex,* it was about finding a part of yourself that had gone missing. And it wasn't about doing something with, or to, someone else—at least it didn't start there. It was about having your *own* experience. It was about re-connecting the wiring of your own sensual vitality—becoming comfortable, physically and mentally, with yourself again.

Of course, you might be tempted to again say: *Easier said than done!* But I know it can be done. This book is based on two principles I strongly believe in:

➤ The sensual aspect is one of the body's systems—just as essential as the circulatory or digestive system—and we need to keep it healthy for the sake of our own well-being.

➤ A person's sensuality and sexuality are best approached in a larger context of her overall fitness level, body awareness, and self-image.

Opening to New Possibilities

It surprised me that someone with a lifetime of expertise in fitness might not feel perfectly at home with some aspect of her body. It soon became clear that physical fitness and the drumbeat of a healthy libido are two separate things. The question was, how to connect the dots?

It became a project: How Kathy Got Her Groove Back. I read the tips in the magazines. Friends dragged me to trendy "cardio-striptease" classes. Meanwhile, I braved a few tentative dates, feeling a mixture of insecurity and resentment at having to go through all this again, at this age.

Finally, I landed in a belly dancing class. And there, at last, I was home! The movement was a revelation—it was tasteful, beautiful, and sensuous. As I watched myself in the mirror, circling my hips, moving my shoulders in ways that were new and challenging to me, I noticed a distinct shift in how I felt about myself—in a word, I felt sexy.

It was *my* moment of opening up to new possibilities.

It took me several months to begin feeling confident in my own femininity and sexual vitality again—to feel both desiring and desirable—and I arrived there through a process similar to the one I'm going to share in this book. I know everyone's issues with sex are going to be different. But whatever yours may be, chances are, the solution comes down to reconnecting with your physical body and tapping back into that inner current of playful sensuality. In other words: *Put the fun back in your body!*

That's what the *Flex Appeal* Program is all about. Through a combination of yoga, dance, strengthening, and flexibility movements, you'll learn to tap into those feelings of vitality and sensuality again—and start feeling sexy, from the inside out. Plus, you'll be getting your body in shape at the same time!

If I had to pick a mantra to guide this process, it would be *open up.* This program will help you do that, and more.

What *Flex Appeal* Can Do for You

This book is for anyone who, for any of a hundred and one everyday reasons, may have drifted out of touch with her body. It will train and condition your body in a way that will help you feel more connected to your physical self in general, and your sensual self in particular.

Two special notes on the program:

- ➤ *Flex Appeal* **is great physical exercise.** This program offers a variety of benefits including strength, flexibility, fluidity of motion, and a more relaxed, expressive body.

- ➤ *Flex Appeal* **is sex appeal** *minus* **the performance anxiety!** There's no need to force the sensual dimension. That's one reason I chose the more fitness-coated term *flex appeal*. This is how I, as a health and fitness expert, interpret the quality that some call sex appeal. If I can simply get you feeling more "in your body," and help you develop a better sensory—and sensual—appreciation of your body, the *sexual* dimension will take care of itself, and will develop in a way that is right and appropriate for you.

A Sensual Disconnect

A friend recently described a workshop she'd attended on "Sacred Sexuality." (This tantalizing idea is a modern offshoot of the ancient Hindu tradition of tantric yoga.) To break the ice, the participants had to say the first word that came to them when they thought about making love. There were many: *connectedness, melting, release, oneness, boundaryless, waterfall, yummy . . .*

My word would be *playful*. This is an aspect of sexuality we sometimes overlook in our culture, for various reasons, but which Eastern philosophies have always understood: Sexual energy is playful energy. En route to my own reawakening, I spent a lot of time thinking about the playful, sensual spirit in our lives—about what causes it to thrive, or to retreat.

I remember back when the feeling of sexual vitality was simply *there*, effortlessly, all the time. That adventure of early womanhood, before career and family took center stage, was a very exciting part of my life.

Time passes, though, and those days give way to practical, survival-oriented concerns. You get busy with your career, you get married, you focus on buying a house and making it a home. You're perpetually short on time, drained of energy; as a result you become less active, perhaps putting on a few pounds, then a few more. Your romantic life succumbs to habit; sex is less frequent, more routine. Meanwhile, you start developing a repertoire of stress-related symptoms such as stomach pains, back pain, or insomnia. Before you know it, you can't get going without your coffee, can't fall asleep without a glass of wine, can't climb to the top of that little hill to watch the sunset. This is how you start to drift out of your body.

Meanwhile, life marches on. Eventually, kids arrive, you hit problems in your marriage, you worry about your aging parents. Maybe you find yourself, as I did, dealing with a physically or mentally ill family member. Suddenly, you're a full-service caretaker.

And what happens? That free, playful spirit—that creative sexual energy that used to dance and sing through your arms, your legs, your hips, your breasts, your smile—begins to fade. Instead of finding expression through your body, it's trapped there and forgotten.

Does any of this sound familiar? Think about how it felt to be first discovering your sexuality. Was there ever a time when your sexuality was fun, unselfconscious, free?

It's almost as though a line is drawn between that free-spirited, sensual enjoyment of the world . . . and becoming a responsible member of society. It's almost as though settling down required *simmering* down.

By the time I hit my late forties, I felt like someone who goes to look up a favorite recipe and finds the page missing. How did I ever create that energy? Would I ever feel that spark, that aliveness, again?

Hot-Wiring the Stalled Libido

Newly single at fifty, I was soon inundated with "empowering" quick fixes from media "sexperts." "Girl, get yourself a good vibrator and a younger boyfriend," a licensed sexologist told me, "preferably about half your age!" I had to laugh. Isn't science wonderful? No problem at all to hot-wire that stalled libido—all it takes is fresh batteries and a boy toy!

Of course, for some women, that might be just the ticket. But for others, such quick fixes don't address the real issue. Most of us, depending on how long we've been out of the water, are not ready to dive into the deep end of our wildest fantasies. We need to start at a more basic level. After all, it's not as if I didn't *know* there were such things as vibrators or younger men in the world. It's just that those approaches—and all the adventurous new things you might try with your husband, if you happen to be married—can take hold only when you first open up to the *possibility.*

It can start small. Maybe a day comes when you look in your dresser and say to yourself: *Okay, this is it, I'm taking all this ratty old underwear that I see every day, that I can hardly wear it's so stretched out, and I'm throwing it all away and buying new stuff.* Then—*then*—you pick out a pair with just a slightly lower cut . . .

And it builds from there. Sure, the first step *might* be that curious-looking "toy" you brought home from your friend's bridal shower. It might be anything. Maybe it was buying this book.

It's about opening up to possibilities.

The key is to find things that *put the fun back in your body.* Because putting the fun back, and putting *you* back, are one and the same.

In the next chapter, I'll describe the parts of the *Flex Appeal* Program and show you why it's such a new and different type of exercise—how it manages to infuse powerful physical conditioning with a spirit of playful sensuality. And why *Flex Appeal* might just be *your* "opening" act.

CHAPTER 2

Flex Appeal— Your Body's Homecoming

The Flex Appeal *Program and How It Works*

DESPITE ITS TITLE, the book you're holding is about much more than just flexibility. My editor and I brainstormed for weeks, searching for the perfect way to describe the total experience of feeling *fit, sexy, and fully alive* in your body. That experience, that elusive "it," springs from a combination of mental and physical qualities, and we settled on *Flex Appeal* as shorthand for a workout that's really one part physical training and one part attitude adjustment.

Playful or cool, dignified or sexy, flex appeal is an aura of ease and self-acceptance. It's that special quality you sense in people who are at home in their bodies no matter what kind of body they have.

The *Flex Appeal* Program

Physically, the *Flex Appeal* Program is something quite new. It's the result of my search for a great strengthening and toning workout that would sculpt and firm the *exterior*, while addressing a woman's inner sensual dimension as well. It's based on my own version of *fluid yoga*—essentially, yoga in motion.

If you want, you can think of *Flex Appeal* as yoga done in a sexy way—or, as a friend of mine likes to say: *Yoga with an ulterior motive.*

What makes fluid yoga sexy is the addition of sensual movement patterns (similar to those I learned in Middle Eastern dance). It's an amazing pairing: Imagine the focus and concentration of a yogi; then add the sensual grace of the belly dancer. That's what we're going for—a strength and flexibility workout that will tickle your libido while it's toning and limbering your body.

Fluid Movement, Strength, and Sensuality

Movement changes everything. The fluid mechanics of *Flex Appeal* bring a new dimension to the yoga poses you'll be doing. You get the basic conditioning benefits of yoga—that is, you'll be getting a great strengthening and flexibility workout—but now you're building:

> ➤ *Fluid* strength

> ➤ *Fluid* flexibility

And in the fluidity, you'll find the sensuality. Although these exercises are not sexual in nature, they are suggestive. They are designed to awaken and stimulate. You might say it's all about *giving your body ideas.*

The great thing is, you don't have to be feeling the least bit sexy to do them. Perform the exercises, and the feeling of sensuality will follow to whatever extent you're comfortable allowing it. It will simply be the natural result of doing these movements.

Fluidity and Fitness

Now it's time for that famous line: *But wait! There's more!* You see, besides helping to stimulate sensuality, the fluid qualities of *Flex Appeal* also provide a totally new and unique type of fitness training.

Your Fluid Body

A healthy body is fluid, inside and out. Feeling 100 percent alive requires the freely circulating flow of movement *and* energy *and* fluids in the body. From the synovial fluid that lubricates our joints, to our spinal fluid, to the water passing through our system and cleansing it of waste products, to lymph fluid and blood—anything that promotes circulation, promotes life.

As we start to get older, though, there's a definite stiffness that seems to creep into the muscles and joints. It's gradual; still, every morning after you've turned forty or so, that walk from the bed to the hot shower seems longer, and the body just a little stiffer, than the day before. By limiting our ability to move freely, this stiffness chokes the flow of energy in our body and limits our sense of aliveness.

This is not just an age thing: I know scores of women in their thirties who—while they may not be creaky in the joints yet—still exhibit this stiffness and the resulting lack of vitality. *Their* longest mile is from the bed to the coffeepot each morning. They're living proof that these blockages of energy, and this lack of flow, can make you *feel* old no matter what your age!

Help can come only through movement. With more than 230 movable and semimovable joints, our bodies have tremendous fluid potential—potential we could reclaim *if* we had a specific system for stimulating it. But until now, that's just what's been missing.

The Missing Slice

If you think of your body's fitness needs as a pie, how would you slice it? I think many active people might slice it two ways at most—into *strength training* (probably with weights) and some form of *cardiovascular work*.

First of all, I love weight training! It's *the* way to maintain strength and muscle mass. Still, I have to laugh at the rigid strut of serious bodybuilders at my gym; their bodies are so unbending. Yes, they've built mass and power, but often at the cost of grace and flexibility.

Likewise, running and other forms of cardiovascular exercise are vital for aerobic health and weight loss. But again, cardio exercise mainly targets only one area of fitness. Serious runners, like serious lifters, develop their own characteristic rigidity in the torso and shoulders.

Our bodies shape themselves according to how we use them. You can usually tell by looking at someone whether she's been spending her time on the track, at the weight rack, or at a desk. It's almost as though we become *lifter-shaped, runner-shaped, desk-worker-shaped, mom-shaped,* and so on.

Can you see what's missing? Weight training and cardio are wonderful forms of exercise. It's great that women today train with these hard-core forms. Still, we largely ignore the body's fluid quality. It's clear we need one more type of exercise in our bag of tricks—something to complement these other forms, while reclaiming the body's fluid potential.

Integration and Flow

At this point, you might be saying to yourself: *Isn't this all just about the need to stretch?* Yes, but it's more than that. The fact is, conventional stretching isn't enough. For one thing, many people's idea of stretching is to do a few token hamstring stretches before working out. Doing a full-body sequence of stretches is better, but it doesn't address your fluid potential because it doesn't involve movement.

Graceful, full-range motion—the kind that treats our bodies like the versatile tools they are—is found in areas of physical training that aim at integration: martial arts, yoga, Pilates, gymnastics, and, of course, dance.

That's why I've constructed my *Flex Appeal* system from two of these forms: *yoga* and *dance.*

YOGA + Sensual Movement Patterns = Flex Appeal

Let's break this formula down and I'll describe why I chose these particular elements.

Yoga—The Foundation of *Flex Appeal*

Of all traditional systems of fitness, none is more directly concerned with improving the limberness of the body than yoga. Yoga recognizes that flex-

All these disciplines can have a place in your plan:

➤ **Weight training** builds muscle mass for shape and symmetry.

➤ **Cardio exercise** burns calories, generates energy and aliveness.

➤ ***Flex Appeal*** creates fluidity, flexibility, and sensuality.

ibility is one attribute you really can improve—and continue to improve throughout your life. From the earliest days of yoga, dedicated practitioners used to astound audiences with their flexibility. Today, yogis in their eighties such as B. K. S. Iyengar and others are often said to have the spines of twenty-year-olds.

In addition to building flexibility, yoga conveys many other benefits also conducive to longevity, as well as to appearance. Yoga tones and strengthens muscle, improves balance, and heightens your sensitivity to your body as a whole. With its emphasis on the breath, yoga can be both energizing and calming. In addition, it teaches you to focus on the moment-to-moment experience of being *in your body*.

From a sensual standpoint, yoga is also unique. I remember my first experiences years ago with a breathing technique called Breath of Fire. After a few minutes, I'd experience a wave of relaxation, openness, and pleasure. Physically, I felt looser, disentangled, calm. Then, in the calmness, I found myself feeling very, very sensual.

For all these reasons, I saw yoga as the perfect foundation for *Flex Appeal*. The next step was to add movement.

The Benefits of Movement and Dance

I described in the first chapter of this book how my *Flex Appeal* journey was energized by my discovery of belly dancing. Since then, I've tried a number of sensual types of dancing—with names like ecstatic dance, trance dance, and shiva. In all of them, I've experienced an exciting sense of freedom and release.

And so the second part of the *Flex Appeal* formula involves sensual movement patterns applied to the yoga poses. While traditional yoga is, among other things, a great form of exercise, a world of sensations opens up when you go beyond the frozen poses and experience how it feels to massage them, so to speak, with movement.

The *Flex Appeal* Workout

The *Flex Appeal* exercises are broken up into four specific areas of the body:

➤ Core and Spine

➤ Hips, Pelvis, and Legs

➤ Upper Body

➤ Face and Head

Each of these areas is introduced through an in-depth routine. These will help you in opening up and decompressing one section of your body at a time. By the time you've worked through these four basic routines, you'll be feeling a sense of fluidity and openness you've probably never felt before. Then you'll be ready to experience three special routines aimed at particular goals. These are:

➤ Fluid Relaxation Meditation

➤ Sensual Strength and Weight Loss

➤ *Flex Appeal* Dance

As you work through each of these, you'll gain greater flexibility and fluidity of movement—*plus* the additional benefits designed into that particular routine.

In chapter 7, *Flex Appeal* Basics, I'll explain in more detail how the routines work, and describe the patterns themselves.

How *Flex Appeal* Unlocks Your Sensuality

The crowning benefit here—besides the physical workout—is that when you move your body in new ways, it changes your sense of yourself. When I do kickboxing, I feel powerful. When I weight train, I feel strong and solid. When I go running in the hills, I feel exhilarated and free. Likewise, when you explore sensual movement, you start to feel more sensual. It really is that simple.

I've proved it to myself: Throughout the course of my exploration of sensual dance, I've felt myself go from, I'd say, a fifty on the sensuality chart to somewhere around a ninety-six! In fact, after several months of working on *Flex Appeal,* I got together with my old belly dance instructor for a refresher. "Kathy, *what* have you been doing?" she asked in astonishment. "Your moves have gotten so fluid!"

It's true, they had. And yours will, too!

The Need for Rejuvenating Exercise

The final reason for the *Flex Appeal* Program is that it provides a means of *recovery* from other, more strenuous forms of exercise. The need for such rejuvenating forms of exercise is too often ignored.

I've found that if I race up the cliffs near my house or do a strenuous track workout, I may need up to four days to recover. If I don't respect this need, I pay for it: I start to notice a heavy feeling in my legs, I'm less alert in meetings, less patient. After decades of feeling consistently energetic, it's strange to have to acknowledge this new fact of life—that one day I can feel like Superwoman, and the next day I feel like I'm ready for the Senior Circuit.

Recovery: Important at Any Age

While it's true that the *amount* of recovery time needed may increase as you get older, the *need* for recovery exists at any age—women in their twenties or thirties are just as likely to overtrain at times. No matter how energetic you feel, pushing too hard for too long has a cost, and yields diminishing returns.

What really brings everything back into focus, physically, is to keep moving, maintain your flexibility, and keep your fluids circulating so that you can be ready to go for that next burst. That's where *Flex Appeal* comes in.

Part II: Your Mind–Body Awareness Project

Now that I've described the *Flex Appeal* workout, let me take a moment to preview the rest of the book.

Remember I said that the sensual movement patterns in *Flex Appeal* were about giving your body *ideas?* The other part of this book deals with being *open* to those ideas your body is getting. To help you open up in this way, I'll be leading you through various topics having to do with the re-connection of the mind and body.

These will include:

➤ Changes that may be happening in your body and life

➤ Disliking your body

➤ Shortchanging your body by being out of touch with its basic energy cycles

➤ Distancing yourself from sensations, especially pleasurable ones

I'll deal with these issues in the chapters that follow:

➤ Chapter 3 discusses the sensual disconnect and investigates some of the reasons you might be feeling less in touch with your sensual side than you used to.

➤ Chapter 4 discusses issues of body image, including develop-ing a nonjudgmental image of your body, what you'd like to change about it, and how to feel better about things you can't change.

➤ **It's fun.** Remember I said the first step in rewiring your sexual vitality was simply to put some *fun* back in your body? The fun of *Flex Appeal* is in practicing the art of moving gracefully and sensually.

➤ **It's powerful.** This is *get-you-sweaty-in-no-time* training, make no mistake—well worth your time from a fitness standpoint alone. You can use this workout to build strength, improve flexibility, and burn calories.

➤ **It's therapeutic.** The stretching and movement challenges in this workout will help you unblock stiff areas of your spine and other joints like nothing else I know. You'll feel relaxed and enlivened.

➤ **It's empowering.** Any strenuous motion is likely to be cathartic, but *Flex Appeal*'s emphasis on the breath (a natural channel for the emotions), and on sensual movement, will help to make it even more so.

➤ Chapter 5 explores the day-to-day ways you may be living outside your body as a result of being inattentive to its needs and cycles, and suggests simple strategies for tuning back in.

➤ Chapter 6 focuses on the five senses, and offers exercises for heightening sensory awareness as a prelude to sensual movement.

What Now?

If you're eager to get started, you can jump now to chapter 7, *Flex Appeal* Basics, and begin learning the exercises. The next four chapters on mind–body issues are meant as a kind of enrichment study, to inspire you to think more deeply about your relationship to your body. They include various self-discovery exercises for you to try. I suggest you work through them at your own pace as you simultaneously begin exploring the *Flex Appeal* routines.

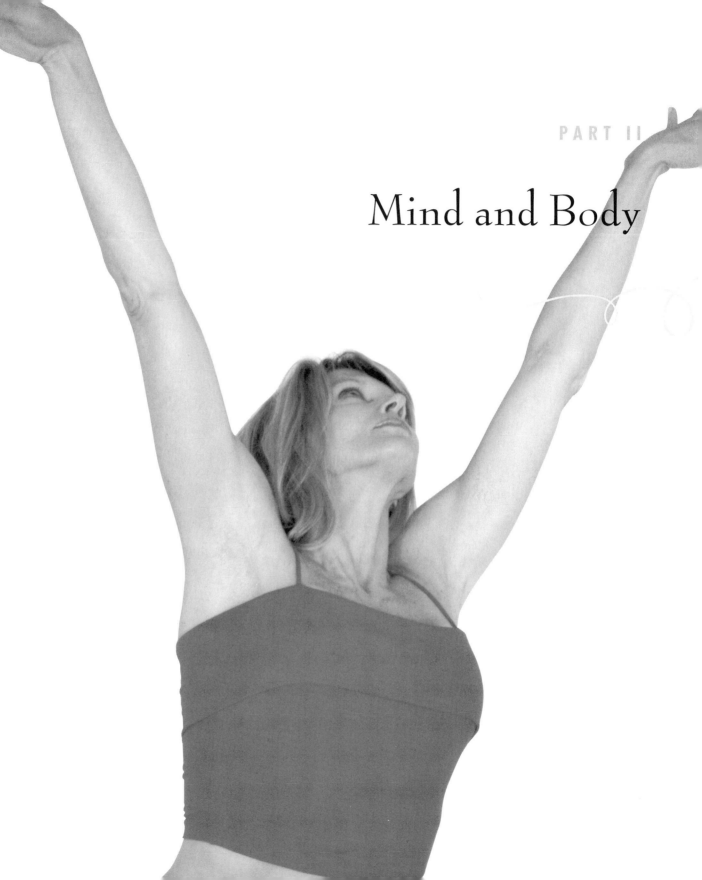

Mind and Body

CHAPTER 3

Life Gets in the Way

Investigating the Mind–Body Disconnect

MANY TIMES when I'm out with my girlfriends, the conversation inevitably turns to the subject of how to keep things fresh with your partner. Whether you've been married fifteen years or are with a boyfriend of one year, it's still the million-dollar question. As I said in the first chapter, though, the deeper issue, the real issue, is how to be comfortable in your own skin. In this chapter, I'm going to talk in more detail about some things that might stand in the way.

Why *would* someone start feeling disconnected from her playful, sensual side? Behind all the euphemisms of *losing your groove, dry spells,* and *missing sparks,* there must be some plain and simple realities. My own story—single at fifty after a stressful separation and divorce—is certainly a common one, but it may not be your situation at all. Other women will have other stories, other paths that have led them to what I referred to in the last chapter as the *sensual disconnect.* So what does it mean?

The *sensual disconnect* means being cut off from the experience of your body. It's not a medical condition; it's just part of the Human Condition.

Another term for it might be *mind–body disconnect*. It's not necessarily age related, although age and physical changes such as pregnancy can play a role. Estrangement from your body may take a variety of forms, including:

> ➤ Disliking your body

> ➤ Being inattentive to your body's natural energy cycles

> ➤ Distancing yourself from sensations, especially pleasurable ones

I realize there are hundreds of possible variations on the theme of being disconnected and, thanks to one or more of them, most of us experience it at some point in our lives.

The Thrill Is Gone, Baby

Most women I've talked to don't have much trouble pointing to the reason they're feeling disconnected sensually. Some find the caretaking aspects of motherhood to be slamming the brakes on a previously active sex life. Others are insecure about changes in their appearance. As one woman wrote to me: "I'm afraid of trying new things in bed. I worry about how I might look in certain positions, and I don't let myself enjoy the experience."

One important question to ask, though, is whether the person was ever connected in the first place. If the disconnection stems from a woman's experience with childhood sexual or physical abuse, for example, then she may not see her sex life slowing down as a problem at all. Many women with a history of abuse are actually relieved to get to a point in their lives where they can focus more on spiritual and health-oriented pursuits, without the emphasis on sexuality or physical intimacy.

Other women with a history of abuse may be actively looking for a way to break through their lifelong ambivalence toward sexual intimacy, in the hope of a deeper connection with their partners and—most important— with themselves. While such a task will require more than just an exercise program, some form of movement therapy may be a part of the trail leading them to a healthier place, with help from a therapist.

But let's say you and your libido are old friends who simply haven't spoken in a while. What about some of the more everyday reasons for experiencing a sensual disconnect?

Nancy's Story

Nancy was single until she was forty-two, when she got married and quickly had twins. Up to that point, she'd always been quite happy with her sexuality. She'd had a lot of men in her life, had never thought about settling down; yet now she's suddenly living in an entirely different universe as a wife and mom of two—a full-time caretaker. At the same time, since her pregnancy, her body has changed in ways that make her feel less attractive. It seems to Nancy that her life has been turned upside down overnight. She's happy with her new connection to her husband and kids, but at the same time, she feels disconnected from *herself*—from all the feelings associated with being that free-spirited single woman. She struggles with what, some days, feels like a tremendous burden, and she laments, "I just want to feel something— some kind of spark inside!" A spark, she says, that she could not only enjoy herself but also share with her husband, to deepen their connection to each other. Nancy is a yoga instructor. Every day, the work of reconnecting to her body is there before her, and every day she takes up the challenge.

Cycles Are Normal

Many of the life events that distance us from our bodies are normal interruptions in a flow of energy that is not always steady but, for most of us, comes in *cycles*.

There are seasons of the year—and of life—when you're full of energy and determination and you want to run and jump and push and grow. There are other times, seasons of stress, when you feel you want to stop everything, circle the wagons, and close in on yourself. When I was going through my divorce, I was physically and emotionally spent. I had no desire for sex—any more than I had a desire for strenuous exercise. Still, twice a week, I would manage to do a very simple regenerative yoga practice. It might only have been a few basic restorative poses, but it was enough to center me and give me the energy to deal with the emotional stress. Equally important, it kept me in touch with my body.

The trouble with many of the normal interruptions in our energy cycles is that they can become permanent if we let them.

A Disconnect Checklist

Generally speaking, the reason behind the sensual disconnect might be any circumstance that has caused you to lose touch with your body. Chances are, in your imagination you're still the sensual and passionate being you always were. Somewhere along the line, something happened to put you off your game. It might have been a traumatic event, such as a death in the family. Or it could simply be that your body isn't feeling, looking, or responding as it used to.

In this chapter, I'll go through some of the normal life changes that can upset the pleasurable relationship with your body.

Excess Weight/Pregnancy/Childbirth

When I was seven months' pregnant and shooting my pregnancy video, I got to talk with other pregnant women about what we were all going through. Half the group were basking in the experience; the other half were thoroughly disgusted with the changes in their bodies and worried that they'd never get back to normal. Many agreed pregnancy had an impact on their sensual life.

For one thing, lovemaking changes when you're pregnant. You're worried about hurting the baby, and it's hard to feel free when you're being so careful. Meanwhile, as your breasts become enlarged and engorged and you put on weight, words like *lustful, sexy,* and *hot* just seem to drop out of your vocabulary. Finally, whatever erotic mystique your body still had is totally lost in the delivery room!

Then, of course, you have the postdelivery fallout—the extra weight gained, the stretch marks (50 to 90 percent of women have them), loose skin that doesn't shrink to its former tautness and tone, and stretched muscles around the vagina. If you underwent an episiotomy, you may have some scarring, soreness, or weakening of the pelvic floor muscles. Not to mention sore nipples from breast-feeding. At this point, *Not tonight, dear* may become a mantra.

Meanwhile, your focus shifts entirely to caretaking. I still remember the first time I tried to bathe my daughter Kate. It was a comedy; she was slipping all over the place and I was frantic, thinking: *Oh my God—this living thing is depending on me to stay alive, and I have no clue what I'm doing!* With all this going on, who can think about sex?

And believe me, a mother of two: If the first child doesn't kill your sex drive, the second one will. After two cycles of pregnancy, diapers, sleep deprivation, breast-feeding, worry, and problem solving, you're looking at five years in which the sex has probably been pretty mediocre. It takes a lot of faith and desire to reverse that trend.

MY TAKE

You definitely lose control of your body during pregnancy. The more okay with that you are, the easier it will be. Many of the physical changes—such as excess weight and sore breasts—are temporary. In addition, exercises to strengthen the pelvic floor (Kegels) can be very effective in helping the muscles around the vagina recover lost tone. The biggest adjustments are in dealing with a new self-image as a mom, and body image as a childbearer. A young mom in my yoga class summed it up when the responsibility of her new role sank in, gasping in shock, *"I can't have sex; I'm somebody's mother!"*

It's truly an all-consuming task for a while. Everyone resents the loss of spontaneity. The questions to ask ourselves, once the time is right again, are: How do we begin to feel sexy again, and how do we revive the playful spirit without it seeming forced?

Hormonal Symptoms/Menopause

Most women report some change in sexual function at menopause. Surveys show that women typically have fewer fantasies, experience poorer lubrication, and may be less satisfied with their partners as lovers. Let's face it: Being constantly draggy, sleep-deprived, and resentful just doesn't mix well with satin and lace.

Plus, there are physical symptoms: When estrogen levels drop, blood supply and secretions decrease, and the vagina doesn't become as wet during sex. The inner walls may become thinner, making intercourse less pleasurable.

Other hormonally related changes that might torpedo a healthy sex life include:

- ➤ Hot flashes
- ➤ Irritability
- ➤ Stress incontinence
- ➤ Complexion problems

The average age of menopause—defined as one year after your last period—is fifty-one. However, the process of going through menopause, also called *perimenopause,* can span as many as five to seven years leading up to that point, during which hormone levels can fluctuate erratically.

MY TAKE

Yes, being on a hormonal trampoline can take a lot of the fun out of your body. For a while, you're crying in the bathroom, wondering why the world just doesn't seem *nice* anymore. But then you start to get some perspective. The consolation, again, is that most of the symptoms are temporary. By coming to understand them better, you start to take control. Right now, at fifty-two, I feel ten times better than I did at forty-five or forty-six. That's because I've figured out ways to sleep better and keep my moods more even, by cutting back on sugar and using meditation and herbs like valerian to unwind.

In the meantime, it's important to communicate very specifically with your doctor about your symptoms. Although hormone replacement carries some risk and is not appropriate for every woman, it can be a godsend in dealing with severe symptoms. For more information, and non-hormonal strategies, see my book *Moving Through Menopause,* and check with resources online such as the North American Menopause Society at www.menopause.org.

Other Physical Problems (in You or Your Partner)

- ➤ Decreased testosterone—a part of normal aging that has been associated with lowered libido and decreased frequency of intercourse
- ➤ Disease or chronic pain, such as low back, gastrointestinal (GI), or neck pain
- ➤ Fatigue
- ➤ Depression
- ➤ Antidepressant medications
- ➤ General stress of work, bills, a new career, and so on

MY TAKE

Some physical problems are more difficult to resolve than others. Chronic depression, pain, or fatigue can be very demoralizing. I don't want to minimize the importance of problems that really call for medical treatment, but I find that physical movement can be useful, by helping change your focus. I also believe that physical exercise can be a way of accessing psychological issues, and that by working with the body—often in a therapy setting—emotional pain can be uncovered and worked through. As for chronic physical pain, the best treatment can often be rejuvenating exercise, like the program in this book.

Lifestyle

- ➤ Being short on time
- ➤ Feeling distracted by pressing life concerns

Time is an issue for all of us. Learning some time-management skills will definitely help you clear time for your sensual life. The key is to make it a priority—work it into the schedule. Once you've done that, the *other* key is to find fun ways to build anticipation, so that your scheduled time doesn't feel stilted.

MY TAKE

I believe in the power of words, and specifically the terms we use to call our loved ones. If, instead of calling your partner by name, you use endearments like *sweetheart* or *angel,* it *sensualizes* the tone of a conversation. In this way, without spending any extra time at it, you convey sensual messages to your loved one and start planting little seeds. Have fun: Come up with a sexy nickname for your partner. Tease each other on the phone. Make a suggestive remark. Drop a hint. It takes so little effort that it's a good way of getting *yourself* interested, too.

Here's another approach: No matter how busy you are, there are inevitably times in the day when you're forced to wait—in line, in traffic, or "holding" on the phone. Spend that time coming up with a pleasurable fantasy: Imagine the scene, the music, the wardrobe, and so on. All the time you're imagining, again, you're getting yourself in the mood.

Personal Inhibitions

➤ Holding beliefs that prevent enjoyment

➤ Negative attitudes about sex based on religious upbringing or bad experiences

"What do you mean, enjoy sex?" one woman remarked to me with a note of disdain. "Why should I enjoy it? That's something men do!" Other beliefs that might stand in the way of greater sensual vitality could include: *My enjoyment isn't important. I'm not attractive enough to enjoy my body. Sex is really not a subject for polite discussion. Sex is not really important.*

MY TAKE

I think it's helpful to take the focus off *sex* and instead think about appreciating your body. How could there be anything negative about enjoying the miraculous capabilities of the bodies God has given us? Many women, for a variety of reasons, may choose not to be in a sexual relationship—and that's fine. Sensual vitality does not necessarily imply sex—it simply implies a heightened, more energized experience of being in your body.

Issues of how you view your body will be considered in chapter 4, Get Real, and Get On with It!

Relationship Issues

A number of issues can arise between partners to deaden sensual excitement. These may include:

➤ **Lurking questions about your partner's feelings about your body, or your sexuality.** A woman wrote to me to say: "I wonder how my husband feels after seeing me give birth to two children. Does he think I look gross after seeing his children born?"

➤ **Partner's body image.** Sometimes when her partner's body starts to change, a woman finds herself having to deal with *his* feelings about his *own* desirability. Even though you may be comfortable with your partner's body, his discomfort can end up creating distance in the relationship.

➤ **Psychological tension with partner.** Nothing kills ardor like anger. Long-standing resentments and unresolved anger are one of the main reasons couples experience a drop in intimacy.

➤ **Familiarity.** Stop the presses! This just in: Relationships often become less exciting as they grow more comfortable.

My husband says he loves me no matter what but I just do not feel
very sexual being overweight. I look at myself and wonder why he
would be attracted to me. Thank God I have such a wonderful
husband who stands by and supports me.

—Kelly, thirty-two, Eugene, Oregon

Sometimes our partners aren't feeling what we assume they're feeling. Recently, I was speaking with a woman and her husband about her years of breast-feeding three children. The woman claimed to no longer view her breasts as anything sexual. "Any erotic power they may have once had is gone," she said flatly. At that point, her husband shook his head, winked at me, and said, "That's what *she* thinks."

What are *partners,* after all? Partners are people joined by a common interest. Partnership ideally means cooperating toward common goals, communicating, trusting, problem solving—all of which provide the context for a sensual life together. It seems obvious that an open exchange with your partner on these subjects is the all-important first step. Talk with each other. Get outside help if you need it. Intimacy is about sharing what is innermost, essential, and secret—that's the risk and the reward.

Beyond the Roadblocks

One of my readers said it very well in a letter to me: "I've found that most people become what they believe." It's true—and that's why it's so important to try to get past any roadblocks we may have erected that are preventing us from enjoying our bodies. Whether you're a forty-six-year-old mother of three or a twenty-eight-year-old professional who's been putting her job ahead of her health, there's nothing insurmountable standing between you and a more playful, fun relationship with your body.

The truth is, how you *feel* about your sexuality, how you *expect* sex to be at this point in your life, what sort of relationship you have with your partner—these, in the end, are the factors that count. Any woman who wants to energize her sex life can do so. Any woman who simply wants to enjoy greater sensual pleasure in her own body—apart from anything sexual—can do that as well. And any woman who simply wants to tone and strengthen her body for the sake of greater energy and improved appearance can, too.

In each case, the openness and desire are all that's needed. And in each case, the *Flex Appeal* Program will be the catalyst.

CHAPTER 4

Get Real, and Get On with It!

Exploring Body-Image Issues

Flex Appeal Is: ✔ *Stretching self-limiting beliefs.*

WHY WOULD a compliment *sting?*

One day, I was hiking with a group of women, talking about exercise and getting in shape, when one of my friends blurted out, "God, Kathy, I wish I had your butt!" I thanked her, but my first reaction was frustration. You have to understand: Nina is a gorgeous and talented woman in her forties, with a very shapely, voluptuous body. I had the feeling that she'd momentarily lost sight of everything she had to offer by fixating on a detail. So I complimented *her* body. And it was as though I'd opened a wound; she overflowed with protest and embarrassment. I finally had to lighten the situation by interrupting and saying, "Nina, it was a compliment. All you're supposed to say is *thank you.*"

This doesn't happen just with women, either. Another time, I told the man I was dating how handsome I thought he was.

"No, I'm not." He winced, and added ruefully: "When I was *twenty,* I was."

For some reason, in his mind, the word *handsome* was reserved exclusively for twenty-year-olds. He could never be handsome again—no matter how attractive I saw him to be!

Self-criticism is poison. Whether it's because our bodies don't meet arbitrary standards of beauty, or because our looks seem to be slipping away with age, people—especially women—become consumed with dislike of their bodies. This dislike, in turn, infects their sense of self-worth.

In this chapter, we'll look at how to feel good about your body at your current stage of life and how to feel good about yourself overall—body, mind, and spirit.

Body Image and Self-Esteem

The connections between how you see your body and your feelings of self-worth are often difficult to untangle.

Body image is part of the larger concept of *self-image,* on which, to some degree, feelings of self-esteem or self-worth are based. Body image is the mental picture you have of your body—your physical appearance, size, and shape—as well as all the baggage that goes with it: all the feelings and judgments.

While it's not the only factor in self-esteem, body image is an important battleground on which the war of self-esteem is waged. Having low self-esteem may make you feel ugly; on the other hand, feeling ugly might make you feel less worthy as a person. This, in turn, might convince you that changing your appearance would make you feel better about yourself again.

The truth is that nothing—whether it's a new nose or a Nobel Prize—can make you feel truly good about yourself if your thinking is distorted in ways that promote self-criticism.

On the other hand, it *is* true that putting in effort and making improvements can give you confidence in yourself, as well as pleasure in seeing the results. Making constructive changes is empowering and can raise self-esteem by giving you a sense of control.

Since having my children, I am not happy with the way my body looks. My hips have gotten bigger and it makes me feel out of place compared to the rest of the world.

— Kimberly, thirty-three, Buffalo, New York

Passing Judgment

At the heart of self-esteem is our capacity to judge—specifically, to judge ourselves. Objective judgments can be helpful: *Math is a struggle for me; I guess I won't go into bookkeeping.* But when we obsess on specific parts of our bodies and actually reject them outright for various reasons, we're left unable to feel good about the whole. This usually happens because:

➤ They don't meet certain ideal standards.

➤ We have a distorted perception of ourselves.

In her book *The Beauty Myth,* Naomi Wolf cited a *Glamour* magazine survey in which 75 percent of women age eighteen through thirty-five believed they were fat, even though only 25 percent were medically over-weight. Such body-image distortion can lead to weight preoccupation, yo-yo dieting, compulsive eating, eating disorders—and, of course, frustration and low self-esteem.

On the other hand, our capacity to judge is not entirely a bad thing. It enables us to look at areas that need improvement and say: *I need to fix this.* Still, there's an all-important difference between looking in the mirror and saying *This hair needs combing,* versus the self-esteem-bashing *I am just a slob.*

Our task:

➤ To find less critical forms of self-assessment—ones that are simply factual and don't cut to the heart of self-worth.

- ➤ To make clear distinctions between what we can change and what we can't.
- ➤ To put energy into changing what we can, while accepting what we can't.

I call this process *Getting Real* and *Getting On with It.*

Body Dissatisfaction:
The Shame of Not Measuring Up

The earliest tale of body dissatisfaction is told in the Bible. In the Garden of Eden, Adam and Eve lived for a long time with perfectly good body images. They were naked, but since they didn't know the difference, it didn't matter. They were healthy, and their physical needs were all provided for.

Then, one day, God finds them hiding in the bushes. It seems Adam and Eve are suddenly ashamed. God had seen this coming. "Who told you you were naked?" He asks.

"It was all over TV," Adam blurts out.

"I saw it in *Elle,*" Eve adds.

Blaming the Media

As young children, we reveled in a body-image paradise as blissful as Adam and Eve's. We saw no reason for shame; we knew only the joy of being

BEAUTY IS IN THE EYE

In parts of Africa, beauty ideals are just as rigid as they are here, but completely reversed. According to a recent article in the *New York Times,* fat is the fashion in Niger, where young girls actually take steroids to bulk up, pop pills to stimulate appetite, and may even fatten themselves on animal feed to compete in beauty contests!

alive. Then came society's messages—first, about modesty; second, about standards of beauty.

Messages about feminine beauty are, of course, dispensed mainly through TV and magazines. The average graduating high school student has spent more hours absorbing those messages on TV than she has spent in school. At the same time, she's been getting most of her information about diet and health from women's magazines, which may contain *ten times* as many weight loss ads and articles as men's magazines.

TV's power to shape standards is awesome and sometimes even bizarre. Supermodel Tyra Banks appeared on a late-night talk show recently. She was commenting on the appearance of another model who had recently shaved off all the hair on her head. "You think that look is ugly because you're not used to it," Banks said. "But I guarantee, if you saw her on television, after a while you'd say: *Hey, I want to look like that!*"

An extraordinary example, but in general she's right. And that kind of power is hard to resist.

IMPOSSIBLE IDEALS

Suppose you—like young women everywhere—were to scan the media for clues on the ideal body. Suppose you started with underwear ads. You'd find, first of all, that you ideally want to be a white female, five feet eight to five feet ten, weighing 110 to 120 pounds or less. You also need large breasts, a hollowed-out stomach, exposed ribs, and a firm, well-rounded butt. Studies show the idealized woman is also 13 to 19 percent below physically expected weight.

Less than 10 percent of women have the genes to pull this off, leaving the rest to bite the bullet of lowered self-esteem. Indeed, one study found that 80 to 90 percent of American women were dissatisfied with their bodies.

Pressure from Everywhere

Girls get messages about body ideals from other sources, too. Studies show that girls who participate in elite competitive sports such as ice-skating, gymnastics, crew, or dance, in which body shape and size affect performance, are more prone to eating disorders. Teasing from a girl's peers can be another big factor. Even well-intentioned parents who encourage their daughter's weight loss efforts may be reinforcing the connection between being thin and having strong self-worth.

Shame over our failure to meet standards of beauty has been with us for generations. In 1953, Alfred Kinsey found that women were actually more embarrassed to talk about their weight than about their masturbation habits or homosexual behavior. And today, according to the Harvard Eating Disorders Center, more than five million Americans have eating disorders—90 percent of them women.

EXERCISE: EXAMINING YOUR HISTORY

Sit quietly and think about the origins of your body image. When did you first start to be aware of your body being different in appearance from those of others? What were some of the first messages you received about beauty standards? What's the first feedback on your own body that you can remember? Was it a comment from your mother or father? Was it a schoolyard taunt? Can you remember how you felt when you realized how others saw you physically?

Getting Real

The first step toward enjoying your body is to cut through any dissatisfaction or distortion and get real about it. In so doing, you can challenge the caricature you've drawn of yourself and draw a more accurate image—one you can feel good about.

Rose's Story

A friend told me recently about her shocking encounter with a full-length mirror.

Rose is a yoga student. Having worked for several years now, she's quite a good practitioner and often tells her teacher how happy she is about changes she's felt in her body. Recently, she and her husband spent a week-end in Las Vegas. Checking into their hotel, she found that their room had a full-length mirror on one wall. While her husband was out, she decided to do her yoga routine in front of the mirror. This was something she'd never tried before and she was excited to see how she would look. She began a pose and, glancing up, was horrified at what she saw. It was not the pure, perfect ideal she saw in her mind's eye. What she saw was the image of a somewhat overweight middle-age woman doing yoga. She was crushed. It didn't look anything like the way she felt, or wanted to feel.

The Beauty of What Is

Rose's long practice of yoga had brought her feelings of self-worth that had nothing to do with physical appearance—and that's great. On the other hand, she had not completely made peace with her body.

What Rose hadn't seen yet was what I call "the beauty of what is": in this case, that a perfectly normal middle-age body, doing yoga well, *can* be beautiful. Sure, it's different from the way her younger teacher might look. Nevertheless, there's beauty in the pose itself, and there's beauty in the care, precision, and control with which Rose performs it. Anyone watching her would see and admire it. But she was too shocked by the sight of her body to see anything else.

Ideally, two things go hand in hand. First, appreciating your body for what it can do, rather than how it looks. Second, making peace with the physical reality so that you can fully enjoy your body without having to hide it. To be able to appreciate the beauty of what "is"—that's the essence of a healthy body image.

Our first step will be to look in the mirror. . . .

Creating Your Physical Inventory

How accurately do you think you see your body? What do you like about it? What do you dislike? In this next section, I'll lead you through an exploration designed to help you see yourself more accurately, while also helping you recognize and befriend any areas of dissatisfaction. (The self-inventory technique described here is adapted from one described by Matthew McKay, Ph.D., and Patrick Fanning in their book *Self-Esteem*.)

Step 1. Roll Call

Begin by writing down short descriptions of the following areas of your body:

Height	*Arms*
Weight	*Hands*
Body shape	*Breasts*
Face	*Waist or belly*
Individual facial features	*Hips*
Eyes	*Butt*
Teeth	*Thighs*
Lips	*Calves*
Skin quality	*Feet*
Hair	*Types of clothing that look good on you*
Neck	*Types of clothing that look bad on you*
Shoulders	*Your overall style*

TIPS

➤ **Be sure to go through the whole list.** I've provided the list above because without it, you might only list body parts you have strong feelings about—the ones you're self-conscious about, were teased about, and perhaps one or two that serve as your token self-compliments (say, "nice ankles"). In so doing, you might be over-looking much of what's good about your body.

➤ **Be honest.** Without analyzing too much, write down a simple capsule description of each area, in the first words that come to you.

Step 2. Rate Your Responses

Now go through your responses and put a plus sign (+) by things you like about yourself, a minus sign (–) by negatives, and a zero (0) by items about which your feelings are neutral. For instance, your list might read in part:

0 *narrow shoulders*   + *look striking with hair up*

– *thin lips*   – *look terrible in dresses*

+ *slender waist*   + *look good in tailored suits with*

+ *flat stomach*   *padded shoulders*

0 *slight overbite*   + *low-cut pants show off lumbar tattoo!*

– *hippo thighs*

+ *long graceful neck*

Review your ratings. How do the pluses and minuses stack up? Are they about even? If so, it shows you have made a fairly large number of negative judgments about yourself. On the other hand, it's possible that your negatives will all cluster around just one area, such as excess weight. Notice, too, how many are emotional, judgment-laden descriptions ("hippo thighs") and how many are purely factual.

Now let's look at some of the possible distortions that may be at work.

FILTERING

If you notice that you have only one or very few specific negative items, and yet you feel generally unattractive, your self-portrait may have been distorted by *filtering* out all the positive things to be said for your body. When you filter out positives, that little pimple on your nose feels like a searchlight, and you're sure it's all anyone is noticing about you. You become like the beautiful woman whose day at the beach is ruined by her focusing on an extra millimeter of fat at her waistband.

NEGATIVE SHORTHAND

There's a human tendency to reduce complex impressions to simple labels. I call this *negative shorthand*. You can spot this easily anytime you catch

yourself beginning a description of your body with the words, *I'm just . . .*
Typically what follows is anything but complimentary or accurate:

➤ *I'm just a fat blob.*

➤ *I'm just a beanpole.*

➤ *I'm a clumsy oaf.*

➤ *I'm such a shrimp.*

➤ *I'm just a moron.*

Labels may be convenient, but we can't afford to be so simplistic about ourselves—especially when the labels are pejorative and lock us into a negative stereotype. All they do is make it more "convenient" to think poorly of ourselves.

GENERALIZATIONS

It's also possible that your body image may be marred by a generally distorted sense of your body size or shape. Notice whether you have recorded feelings such as "too tall," "too heavy," or "really short." These are value judgments based on foggy thinking. How tall are you in inches? How tall is too tall? Who says so?

Step 3. Revise Your Self-Portrait

Now it's time to revise your list to create a more accurate image—and, if you're willing to stretch your mind, a more positive one. This next step may sound a little far-fetched, or like too much work. The truth is, it can be surprisingly instructive. If it sounds like fun, try it. If not, read through and simply *imagine* doing it—maybe you'll get curious and want to try it for real.

Begin by taking several large sheets of newsprint or strips from a roll of butcher paper and taping them to the wall. They should cover an area at least as wide and high as your body. Remove as much of your clothing as is convenient; then, with your back to the wall, trace your body with a wide-tipped marker. Trace as close to your body as you can for accuracy. (With a

We're very influenced by the spin that words put on ideas. Advertisers and political speechwriters understand this and carefully craft the "positioning" of their products and the "angle" of their stories. How you spin your own self-concept is central to how you feel about yourself.

➤ Being *timid* is bad, but being *risk-averse* is smart.

➤ A *workaholic* is bad; a *go-getter* is good.

➤ Being an *exhibitionist* is bad; being *the life of the party* is good.

➤ Being *old-fashioned* is bad; being a *traditionalist* is good.

➤ *Scatterbrains* are a pain, but *spontaneous creative types* are fun.

When all else fails, resort to French: After all, *bon vivant* sounds so much better than *goof-off!* The same principle applies to physical descriptions. Why not . . .

➤ A *generous* nose instead of a *big* nose.

➤ *Luscious* instead of *flabby.*

➤ *Voluptuous* instead of *heavy.*

➤ *Athletic* instead of *flat-chested.*

Think about the words you use to describe various aspects of yourself. Are they the words that create appeal, or words that downgrade? Never underestimate the power of the words you choose!

---

little care, you can do this by yourself, although you might find it easier to do this exercise with a friend.)

The impact of the tracing comes from the fact that it's not the familiar mirror reflection that we look at every day without really seeing. The traced image is novel. It doesn't move; therefore, it allows you to step back and view it objectively.

Now spend some time looking at the proportions of your body tracing. That's you! Does it seem "too" anything? What impression would you have of a person with this shape? Would it be the same you've been carrying of yourself? Or does it seem like a reasonable size and shape for someone to be?

Next, with your list in hand, revise your negative items, this time writing your comments directly onto your image on the wall.

Remember, the problem lies not in having weaknesses or flaws; as McKay and Fanning point out, the problem is in "the ways in which you use your weaknesses for destructive self-attacks." So this time, try to find ways to describe your weaknesses nonpejoratively, without disparaging or downgrading.

Here are some guidelines for revising your negatives:

> Remove negative-sounding adjectives like *ugly, flabby,* and the like. These words are like tiny pebbles in your shoe.

> Remove terms of taste and opinion and replace them with objective descriptions: Instead of *too tall/too curly,* for instance, write *5'10"/tightly curly hair.*

> Don't be dramatic: "My skin looks like I've been living in a cave."

> Don't be vague: "My legs are in bad shape."

> Alternatively, ask yourself how someone who *liked* the attribute would describe it.

CHECK YOUR BAGGAGE

How many of the items on your list *seem* objective but are actually thinly disguised traps of judgment? Think about what assumptions might underlie these factual descriptions. Maybe you would describe yourself, very factually, as having small breasts. On the surface, it's just a fact: They're small, and that's fine. But what beliefs and preconceptions about breast size are working on a subconscious level to make you feel dissatisfied with this fact? If you were to consciously examine the question, do you honestly believe that larger breasts make a woman significantly happier—or smarter, funnier, wiser, or more lovable? Or that *anything* external, for that matter, has that much power over whether a person can live a satisfying, successful life? I'm not naive; I'm not dismissing the social leverage that often comes with being attractive. What I'm saying is that subconscious assumptions develop far too much power over our thoughts if they remain unexamined. (A recent study actually showed a higher rate of suicide among women who'd had breast enhancement, suggesting that obtaining a desired breast size did not bring happiness to the very women who'd believed that it would.) So open up that baggage and see if you can't lighten the load.

Step 4. List Your Body's Strengths

Now add some strengths to your image on the wall. Write positive messages about different parts of your body and what they can do. "Killer tennis serve." "Great kisser." If you're a perfect spoon-fit with your partner, or a good tree climber, write those down.

Once you've finished, spend some time rereading and thinking about your descriptions, and absorbing the whole picture that's emerging.

Getting On with It:
Seven Habits of a Healthy Body Image

1. Set Realistic Goals

As we get older, we may occasionally compare ourself to the twenty-year-old in our memory and fall short—like my male friend at the beginning of this chapter. Meanwhile, the twenty- or thirty-year-old may look at *her* body and feel dissatisfied or ashamed because it's not sufficiently thin, tall, curvy, lean—or any number of ideals. That's why your first step has been to look truthfully at your body, without judgment or self-criticism.

I feel sexier and more alive as a fifty-two-year-old than I ever have before. Those years of experience have taught me who I am, where my power is, and how to use what I've got.

My idea of a realistic goal is this: *I want to look and feel good for my age and for the basic type of body I have.* That means focusing on vitality, fluidity, and freedom of movement, more than on absolute strength or ideal weight.

2. Take Charge of Things You Can Change

Any changes you make to your physique will always be relative to your basic body type. Whether you are a long and narrow *ectomorph,* a soft and curvy *endomorph,* or a muscular and athletic *mesomorph,* your basic shape will remain as you become heavier or leaner versions of it. Likewise, if your tendency is to store fat above the waist in the classic "apple" shape, that will remain true however little fat you have. Same with "pears," whose fat is stored below the waist.

There are many aspects of your body you *can* change, though, to improve your appearance and your well-being:

- ➤ Muscle-to-fat ratio
- ➤ Posture
- ➤ Muscle tone
- ➤ Core strength
- ➤ Fluid movement

To a degree, you can also improve body proportions by working to develop the muscles in areas that seem naturally underdeveloped—for example, developing more muscle in your shoulders to balance out naturally wide hips.

WEIGHT LOSS

The issue of excess weight deserves a footnote in light of the unrealistic ideals of thinness I talked about earlier. On the one hand, we do have in our society an unhealthy obsession with being thin. Studies show that by age ten, half of girls surveyed were dissatisfied with their bodies, and specifically wanted to be thinner, while 40 percent of fourth graders reported that they diet either "very often" or "sometimes." On the other hand, we also have an epidemic of obesity: Between 1963 and 1991, the rate of childhood obesity *tripled,* from 11 to 35 percent.

The healthiest course, as always, is moderation. A few extra pounds aren't a problem, but thirty, forty, or fifty extra pounds can have serious health consequences. Overcoming obesity is not an issue of self-esteem, it's an issue of self-preservation.

I suggest you don't spend one more minute of your life worrying about the "last ten pounds." Just do what you can through reasonable efforts at a healthy lifestyle, and congratulate yourself on a job *well enough* done. Then get on with enjoying life!

3. Adapt to What You Can't Change

How do you make peace with less lovable body parts? First, realize that the problem is not the feature itself; the problem is that it bothers you. Here are some techniques for changing your perspective.

EXERCISE: RESIZING

Remember in the Edgar Allan Poe story "The Telltale Heart," how the faint sound of the murdered man's heartbeat seemed to get louder and louder until the culprit went mad? This is a good example of things taking on exaggerated significance.

If you seem to be blowing things out of proportion—suck them back down to size!

An NLP (neurolinguistic programming) technique that works well for some people is this: Relax, close your eyes, and breathe comfortably for a moment. Imagine the feature that bothers you. See it clearly in your mind. Make the picture as vivid and real as you can—see it in a real setting, with specific sounds and lighting and associated details. Now begin to see a box around the scene, like the frame around a picture. Imagine the frame shrinking, and watch the picture shrink as the frame closes in. Make it smaller, smaller, smaller, until it seems miles away and the sounds are lost in an echo, as at the bottom of a well. Imagine it continuing to shrink until— poof!—it vanishes. Immediately call to mind a happy memory, with all its associated details. Fully see this happy scene in vivid color, filling the screen in your brain. Now smile broadly and open your eyes. Practice this visualization regularly.

EXERCISE: CELEBRATING IT

One of the most liberating techniques I've discovered is to actively celebrate the part of your body you don't like. If you can make that part of you seem lovable, it may just become more lovely.

Unless you're in a group of women all trying this together, you'll want to do this exercise when you're alone. The idea is to put the body part on display nonverbally—using gesture and body language—and experience how it feels to do so. Exaggerate it. Thrust it forward. Flaunt it. Put on some music and do a dance featuring it. Be bold with it and make the universe acknowledge it.

EXERCISE: CREATING YOUR OWN (VIRTUAL) COMMUNITY

Think of ways to create a setting that normalizes your body. For example, create a collage of photos of people who look like you. Find photos of nonmodels, of "real people." Cut photos out of newspapers or out of your church bulletin. The Web can also be a source of photos. Crazy as it sounds, you can actually do a Web search for "big noses" or "small breasts" or "Rubenesque body" and you'll often find images to choose from. (I recommend doing this with your search engine set to exclude explicit images.) You'll even find, in some cases, other people "celebrating" the body trait you deplore.

By doing this, you can become your own media source in the cause of beauty diversity: Flood your brain with images of normal people who look just like you. Take back the airwaves!

4. Focus on Function

Focus more on what your body can do than how it looks. By doing so, you free yourself from the opinions of others. At the same time, you discover a treasure trove of qualities that can't be tarnished by age: energy, sensuality, confidence, vibrancy, capabilities, and skills—all of which have their own allure. Train yourself to see the functioning of your body for the miracle it is, and take pride and pleasure in the sum of who you are.

EXERCISE: WHAT I LIKE ABOUT MYSELF

Write down five things you like about your body. These can be functional or aesthetic. Then write down five things you value about yourself as a person. These can include skills, abilities, talents, qualities, or accomplishments. Do you find it hard to identify positive things about yourself? Read this list aloud to your partner or to a friend. (Adapted from *Promoting Healthy Body Image: A Guide for Program Planners,* published by Best Start, Ontario, Canada.)

5. Look Beyond Your Body

As often as possible, widen your awareness beyond your body. Think about all the things you enjoy doing that don't involve food or losing weight. What things give you pleasure as you go through your day? Start a list of activities you enjoy doing, adding to it whenever you discover a new one. How many of these things do you really allow yourself to do frequently? What stops you from doing them more often?

EXERCISE: TAKE A RISK

Make a list of things you'd like to do in your life but are afraid of doing. Then ask yourself what stops you from doing these things. Identify one thing you think you might be able to accomplish in the next few weeks. List the steps you'd need to follow to achieve it. Tell a friend about this exercise and promise to report back after several weeks to tell her what you've done.

6. Stop the Ranting and Rating

It's human nature to make judgments, but some women seem to make a profession of it. Wherever they are, whatever they're doing, their conversation is all about judging everyone and everything around them. *That girl has a great body. Hers isn't so great. Look at her. Who? With the big boobs. What is that she has on?* (And so on.)

This mind-set is corrosive. First, it tremendously limits your experience: When you're focused on appearance, it's all you see. Second, it's impossible not to turn these judgments inward and start to rate yourself on that same value scale. *My lips aren't as full as hers. My teeth aren't as white.* Begin the comparison game, and you'll never measure up.

There's so much to appreciate besides the fact that the girl next to you has a great body. For heaven's sake, who cares? Notice it, but don't dwell on it. You have to stop judging others so you can stop judging yourself.

7. Take Charge of Your Environment

Because my work involves photo and video shoots, I need, at times, to be especially conscientious about my appearance. Nevertheless, I try to separate the world I *work* in from the world I *live* in. In particular, I'm very aware of the attitudes about appearance among people I spend time with.

If you hang around with people who are always talking about appearances—with men who view women as "arm candy," or women who can only talk about other women's clothes and bodies—it's hard not to either (a) buy into this very limited view of life, or (b) feel cut off from other parts of yourself.

I personally love being around people who involve themselves in the world of ideas—of art, politics, charity work, and so on. I find their wider perspective stimulating, but the main reason I enjoy it is that it allows me to be more fully myself. When I'm with people who take a broader view of the world, I feel that I'm being appreciated for all I have to offer.

A Final Thought: Taking Life Off Hold

How many personal goals have you postponed until the day you have the ideal body? Too often, we sacrifice great pleasures in life by clinging to obsessive ideas about our appearance.

Take a tip from my friend Natalie:

Natalie's husband bought her a two-piece swimsuit before a trip to Europe. She was aghast; never in her dreams would she have picked out such a thing. Bravely, she packed it. Then she got to the beach in France and saw all these *bodies*—big, small, fat, thin, cellulite-dimpled; flat chests and huge chests, sagging breasts, poochy stomachs—a panorama of normal, wonderful human variety and imperfection. She hopped into her two-piece and joined in.

You, too, can make that decision—to shrug off the illusion of perfection and let yourself enjoy life in the body you have.

CHAPTER 5

Getting Back in Your Body

Honoring Your Body's Energy Cycles

Flex Appeal Is: ✓ *Opening up lines of communication between your mind and body.*

I N THE FIRST CHAPTER, I said one of our goals would be to rediscover how it feels to be sensually alive and in your body.

What does it mean to *be in your body*? We've already looked at the issue of body image; certainly, acceptance and appreciation for your body are key to feeling more alive in your skin.

Another aspect of this experience has to do with how connected you are to your body's physical workings—specifically, to the cycles that represent your most basic needs for sleep, food, exercise, recovery, and so on. Learning to understand and honor these cycles is another step back "into" your body.

A healthy relationship with your body is something you reinforce with dozens of individual choices every day.

Spotting the Patterns

All aspects of our well-being flow in cycles. Yet I'm always surprised when someone hasn't figured out her own energy rhythms—when she hasn't noticed, for example, what time of day her body is most "ready" for exercise, critical thinking, creative work, sex, sleep, and so on. Coming to terms with your energy cycles is one of the most basic levels of body awareness, and can be done only by observing your body.

When people ask me the secret to living fully in their bodies, I tell them honestly: It's all about trial and error—especially error! It's about learning to *spot the patterns.* It took me years of being on the road, with the stress of travel and performance, to learn exactly what I need to do to keep myself going at my peak.

For example, I've had several times in the past month when my glands were a little swollen. Now, that's a small thing, sure. But I've learned (the hard way) that it's something I need to listen to—it tells me I'm under extra stress. By being sensitive to the small things, I can adjust my life in small ways to keep myself healthy.

It takes time to spot the patterns that hold clues to your well-being. But this is how you live *in* your body, rather than in spite of it. Think about your own patterns as we work through the topics in this chapter.

Energy Cycles and Rhythms

How much thought have you given to your body's energy cycles throughout the day, the month, and the year?

Daily Cycles and Your Body Clock

You're probably familiar with the terms *larks* and *owls,* and probably know someone (maybe even yourself) who fits the classic description of a morning or night person. Truth is, though, most of us are not extreme larks or owls, but fall somewhere in the middle. If left to our natural rhythm, we tend to rise somewhere between 7 and 8 A.M., get sleepy around ten at night, and fall asleep by midnight, with variations of up to an hour or two either way.

More important is the fact that, whatever hours we keep, we tend to follow a consistent pattern of energy and bodily function over the course of the day. This inner clock is governed by chemical processes in the human body that synchronize themselves to the light–dark cycle of the environment. Coming to terms with your cycle will help you in everything you do.

If you took your temperature every four hours around the clock, you would probably find that it rose and fell by a few tenths of a degree over a twenty-four-hour period. You'd also find that the periods of higher temperature would correspond with periods of higher energy and mental alertness, while the dips in temperature would correspond with sleep, or with that slump period during the day when you feel the need to rest and recharge.

The standard energy cycle for most of us is:

Upon waking:	*Body temperature and metabolic rate rise; sex hormones at their peak.*
Midmorning:	*Highly alert. Best time for activities requiring critical thinking and concentration.*
After lunch, early afternoon:	*Energy and alertness plummet as body temperature drops. For many, an afternoon nap is a refreshing, natural response.*
Mid to late afternoon:	*Body temperature and energy rise again. Mental faculties return.*
Late afternoon:	*Metabolic peak; a good time to exercise and then eat dinner.*
After dinner, about two hours before bed:	*Energy and metabolism drop, melatonin levels rise, preparing us for sleep.*
Pre-dawn:	*Deep sleep; body temperature is at its lowest. Studies show that most one-vehicle accidents, as well as industrial shift worker accidents, happen during this period.*

Most of us have an intuitive sense of our energy profile. Still, it's uncanny how we try to fight it—to work, eat, or drive when we should be sleeping; or, conversely, to squander our most valuable brain time on activities that could easily be done during less alert periods.

Knowing and, more importantly, *respecting* your body's daily energy map is a great way to make yourself more productive, improve the effectiveness of exercise, reduce the likelihood of accidents, improve your sexual performance, and, in general, increase your enjoyment of life.

Mismatched Couples

How to cope with a mismatch between your body's energy cycle and that of your mate can be a huge challenge. Out-of-sync schedules cut down on shared activities and reduce the sense of intimacy. Sometimes, resentments flare up if the mismatch leaves one partner feeling he or she is being avoided. Researchers at Brigham Young University found that mismatched couples were four times more likely to argue or report other marital difficulty. The solution is to work extra hard at creating a sense of togetherness; this takes a lot of compromise and creative problem solving. My advice: Lark-versus-owl compatibility is an important factor to look at *before* entering a serious relationship!

Yearly Cycles: Don't Fight 'Em

I've noticed that my energy and motivation are very seasonal. Calendar landmarks like the beginning of school, the advent of spring, and the long days of summer are all times when I feel a surge of energy and a desire to be active.

In contrast to these high-energy times, I go through high-stress times around the winter holidays and the end of the school year. During these periods, it's all I can do to squeeze in a brief daily yoga practice or walk.

Experience has taught me not to fight my cycles, but rather to expect them, and flow with them. This means taking the emphasis off intensity and just focusing on consistency. Otherwise, I find myself fighting the natural rhythm of my body, trying to push when I haven't the time or energy. The result is always a crash landing, pangs of guilt, and a longer down

I never recommend skipping a workout just because you're feeling low-energy. On the other hand, fatigue might indicate overtraining or a compromised immune system. That's why I suggest what training expert Jerry Robinson calls the Ten-Minute Test. On those days when you *want* to work out, but you think you might be feeling a little dizzy, or fluish, or sleepy, simply start your workout and give it all you've got for ten minutes. Then check in with your body: Are you feeling better or worse from the exercise? If you can't honestly say you're feeling better, stop. Your body probably needs a day off. But don't skip your workout just because you're tired.

phase than I would have had if I'd staged a controlled descent. Truly an out-of-body experience to avoid!

Sleep

As with most body needs, good sleep doesn't just happen; it takes self-observation and awareness to spot obstacles to what the Irish proverb calls "the best cure in the doctor's book."

We all *sleep*, but we don't all get the rest we need. A 2001 survey by the National Sleep Foundation found that 63 percent of Americans are chronically sleep-deprived. I have to tell you: Sleep is one of my favorite things in the world, and I put a lot of importance on trying to get it right. Here are some techniques I've collected that may help you do the same.

Exercise and Sleep

Exercise is a double-edged sword when it comes to sleep. Initially, exercise has an energizing effect, which then gives way several hours later to a greater sense of relaxation. Research shows that afternoon exercise can promote deeper sleep at night; on the other hand, exercising less than three hours before bedtime may keep you awake. Try doing your afternoon exercise five to six hours before bedtime.

To Nap or Not to Nap

Most sleep experts agree that the urge to sleep during the day indicates some degree of sleep deprivation. Napping is an excellent way to make up the debt, and can promote alertness if you need to work or drive. Regular napping, however, can perpetuate the cycle by making it harder to doze off at night. An afternoon power nap of twenty minutes or less is fine, but if you want to improve nighttime sleep, don't go beyond that.

Nighttime Hydration

Believe it or not, your body loses as much water asleep as awake. Still, drinking large amounts of fluids before bed is likely to disturb your sleep through trips to the bathroom. The solution is to stay well hydrated all day long, and taper off on fluids during the hours just before bedtime.

Alcohol at Bedtime

The evening nightcap, however popular, is not a habit endorsed by sleep specialists. While a small amount of alcohol may help put you to sleep, experts say it makes for a less restful sleep through the night—especially during the periods of deep sleep just before morning. You may feel that you've slept, but you won't be well rested.

Caffeine Sensitivity—Fine-Tuning It

If you love coffee, you're probably not going to give it up. But consider this: Caffeine sensitivity varies greatly, so even if you follow the standard recommendation and avoid caffeine before bedtime, your insomnia could still be caffeine induced. Some people are too revved up to fall asleep *ten to twelve hours* after their midmorning coffee break. The only way to gauge your body's sensitivity is to give up caffeine altogether for at least a week, then reintroduce it and notice the effects. Start by restricting it within six hours of bedtime and work backward if necessary.

Tips for a Better Night's Sleep

- ➤ If you often awaken with a sore throat or dryness in your nose, try using a humidifier.
- ➤ Avoid spicy foods, and large meals in general, within three hours of bedtime.
- ➤ The bedroom? Three words: *dark, quiet, cool*—especially cool. Studies show that a too-warm bedroom is more sleep disrupting than either noise or light.
- ➤ Develop a way to wind down before bed. Start by disconnecting from any stimulating activity at least an hour before you retire. Then take a hot bath, give yourself a foot rub, or read a relaxing book. Unburden your mind by writing in your journal, meditating, or praying.
- ➤ Be consistent about bedtime, but if you don't fall asleep within fifteen minutes, get out of bed until you're sleepy enough to try again.

Appetite and Nutrition

Eating when you're hungry, stopping when you're full—it sounds so simple! Nevertheless, appetite is a prime area where people fall out of sync with their bodies.

Ignoring Hunger

For me, one of the big challenges of life is maintaining a steady energy level with regular meals and healthy snacks. My body is very particular about this; if my food intake is a little off, my energy will plummet and I become much more susceptible to the lure of sweets or caffeine. It's taken me years to understand and perfect my eating habits.

What stops *you* from being in touch with the truth about your food needs? How many times this week did you experience hunger pangs? Skip a meal? Eat in the car? Snack instead of eating a full meal? Feel light-headed or other symptoms of low blood sugar? How many times a month do you experience gastric symptoms such as stomach pains, gas, or bloating?

EXERCISE: HUNGER AWARENESS

Using a food diary form like the one below, try to spot the patterns in your eating habits and experiment with small changes. Do you shortchange your food needs because you're rushed, stressed, or worried about your weight? Try establishing a regular schedule of more frequent, smaller meals and record your body's response.

Sample Food Diary page:

Date / Time	Hunger Level (1–5) (1=lowest, 5=highest)	Food Eaten	How did you feel afterward?

Notice the connection between your decision to eat and your hunger level. Are you always pinning your appetite meter before you give in to those hunger pangs? Also, notice how various foods affect you afterward.

Emotional Eating

Then there's the other side of the eating spectrum. How often do you finish food so it doesn't go to waste? Eat food without tasting it? Down a quantity of food (say, a full bag of Oreos) without realizing it until afterward? How often do you take second or third helpings, even though your stomach is uncomfortably full? How often do you eat to calm your nerves?

If you are an emotional eater, one who often turns to food for comfort rather than sustenance, it may be hard to train yourself out of it without professional support; however, one technique that may help is to spread out your daily calorie allowance into four meals instead of three. I tend to be a bit of a nervous eater myself; often, it's the *sensation* of eating that I'm really looking for. I find it works well for me to eat four-hundred-calorie meals at intervals of 7 A.M., 11 A.M., 4 P.M., and 7 P.M. This way, I get the enjoyment of eating more frequently without a lot of extraneous snacking.

Tips for Dealing with Appetite

➤ Design your own healthy, self-nurturing ritual to take the place of unnecessary eating. For instance, it might be to make a cup of tea and read a single chapter from the latest *Harry Potter*. It might be to sequester yourself in the bathroom for a steamy hour-long spa session, complete with fragrances and music. Or take a walk to a compelling destination such as a park or a friend's house.

➤ Fill up on water. Studies show that a glass of water can stop food cravings in most cases.

➤ Put cravings on a ten-minute delay. Often, you can wait them out.

➤ Try high-intensity exercise such as kickboxing or dancing— something that offers an emotional release.

➤ When all else fails, see a counselor or therapist who specializes in eating problems.

Personal Nutrition

At this point, everyone's well versed in the standard nutritional canon. A balanced diet, a moderate calorie intake—these we know (even if we don't always follow them). But there's another important aspect of good nutrition, which is learning the specifics of your own *personal* needs. What's your personal premium-grade fuel?

Over the years, I've learned some important lessons from my body. For instance, as a classic morning person, I know I need to start the day with a good, high-octane breakfast. What I've *learned* is that it makes a huge difference what I eat. I've found that it has to be protein or whole grains, and that I absolutely need to stay away from refined carbohydrates and sugar. As high as my energy is in the morning, if I start out the day with pancakes and maple syrup, I'll be back in bed before lunchtime.

It can take years to learn your unique nutritional needs through random experience, and even then you may only notice the big problems—the oysters that gave you hives, for instance. If you want to optimize your nutritional awareness, the fastest way is to keep a food diary for a few weeks and note all the changes in mood and energy level that occur with different foods.

Water and Weight Loss

We all know the importance of water to bodily function. What you may not know is that drinking water is important for weight management as well. According to researchers, the thirst mechanism is often mistaken for hunger, leading to unnecessary eating. One glass of water was enough to silence midnight hunger pangs for almost 100 percent of the dieters in a University of Washington study. Interestingly, feeling bloated due to water retention, far from being a signal to drink less, is a sign of extra sodium in your body and, surprisingly, can best be reduced by drinking *more* water to help flush it out.

According to a recent survey, only one in five of us meets the famous recommended quota of eight glasses of water a day. Three-quarters of Americans don't drink enough to avoid dehydration, and 9 percent of those surveyed said they didn't drink any water at all. Given that water makes up more than 70 percent of the solid tissue in our bodies, including muscles and bones, you can't get much more out of touch with your body than that!

Here are some more water tips:

➤ Your body loses as much water asleep as awake.

➤ You need as much water in cold weather as in warm weather.

➤ Don't wait for thirst to remind you to drink—but if you do feel thirsty, don't delay.

Exertion, Overtraining, and Recovery

Over the years, I've noticed a particular type of mind–body disconnect among those of us who love to exercise. It's the feeling that, to be fit, you always have to be overloading and pushing through the pain. Years ago, when I was teaching aerobics, I'd pour on everything I had and then be so weak afterward I'd collapse. It turned out I was anemic; my doctor was amazed that I could get out of bed, let alone teach. It sounds crazy, but I was driven; I felt that if I couldn't move and expend energy, something was wrong. One day I ended up on the curb crying because I couldn't run as hard as I thought I should.

I finally realized that it's okay to take a day off. In fact, it's essential. There's a time to go for broke, and there's a time to recover.

Recovery doesn't mean that you do nothing. Instead, I recommend some form of what I call *rejuvenating* exercise. Pick something less de-manding of your energy that still provides a challenge to your muscles. As I mentioned in chapter 3, this is one of the purposes of *Flex Appeal*—to help maintain alignment, flexibility, circulation, and, to some degree, muscle tone during periods of recovery.

Flex Appeal is designed to work as a regenerative routine, as well as a power routine. Check chapter 12 for the sequence called Fluid Relaxation.

Things to Watch For

If you're not making the progress in your training that you once were, and you find you're often fatigued, it's time to consider taking a break. Other symptoms of overtraining include loss of appetite, weight loss, muscle twitching or shaky hands, poor sleep, frequent colds, and an elevated resting pulse rate.

Overtraining Rx

In cases of serious overtraining, start by taking a week off (or two) to let your body recover, then cut back on the number of workout days per week, the number of exercises, and the number of sets.

For milder cases of overtraining, substitute more rejuvenation exercise such as yoga, stretching, or easy walking until you're feeling energetic enough to resume your normal schedule.

Physical Pain

The first response most of us have to physical pain is, of course, *Make it stop!* This often leads us straight to the medicine cabinet—screening out the pain, but also obscuring its cause.

Pain is important information. Medication may be the best course *after* you've listened to the pain and determined the problem. My approach to pain is to become a detective. What's triggering it? What happens if I change this or that aspect of my workout? Can I get rid of this headache with a large glass of water? Can I work the soreness out of my joints by stretching them? Pain is just another sensation that helps us maximize our relationship with our body.

Sexual Rhythms

The idea of sex should ideally make you feel excited and aroused; afterward, it should leave you feeling satisfied and relaxed. If this isn't what's happening, it might be an issue of timing.

Synchronizing the timing of your lovemaking to the cycles of your body—and to those of your partner—is something of an art. Suppose, for instance, you're the type that feels supercharged after sex; a single orgasm never feels like enough, and your body is so full of vibrating energy afterward that sleep is impossible. Meanwhile, your partner is ready to roll over and say good night. In this case, a morning session would probably be more satisfying for both of you. He'll have more energy and willingness to extend the session, and you'll have a place to channel your postsex energy by transitioning into your day.

In general, it's not a good idea to push your body into having sex if you're not feeling like it. If you're overtired or tense, you're probably not going to enjoy yourself, and you'll only set a bad precedent. Better to wait for a time when you're feeling rested and receptive.

Of course, I can just hear some wives saying: "In whose world does *that* work? My husband is constantly wanting sex when I'm too tired." If that's true, it may be that you and he simply have different levels of desire. This can be stressful, but can be worked out if you're both willing to compromise.

DIFFERENT LEVELS OF DESIRE

If you and your partner have very different levels of desire, the trick is to figure out how to balance one person's need for satisfaction with the other person's need not to feel pressured. According to David Osborne, Ph.D., a psychologist at the Mayo Clinic, one possible compromise involves the partner with the lower level of desire being willing to provide sexual satisfaction in ways that don't involve sexual intercourse. This frees that person to participate without feeling any pressure to become aroused if he or she doesn't wish to. In many cases, this relieves the tension of the situation and you *both* may end up enjoying yourselves more.

Here's something else to consider: Testosterone—the hormone of male sexual arousal—is in peak production in the early-morning hours. Likewise, circadian energy rhythms impact on sexual arousal. Simply finding

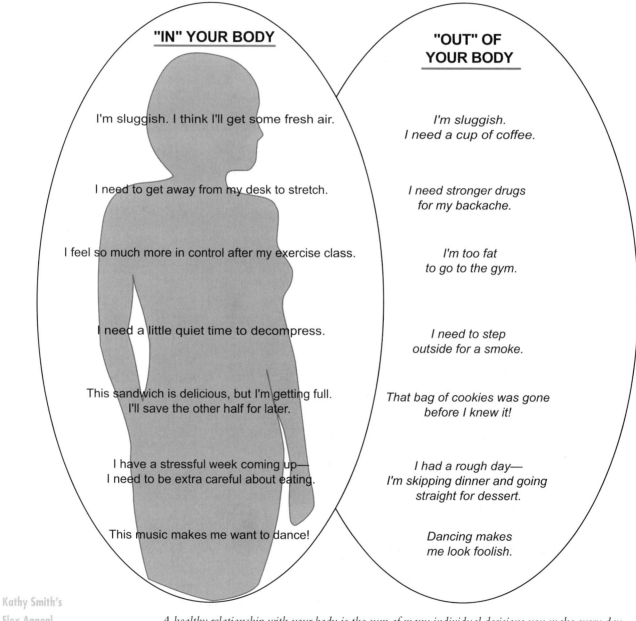

"IN" YOUR BODY

I'm sluggish. I think I'll get some fresh air.

I need to get away from my desk to stretch.

I feel so much more in control after my exercise class.

I need a little quiet time to decompress.

This sandwich is delicious, but I'm getting full.
I'll save the other half for later.

I have a stressful week coming up—
I need to be extra careful about eating.

This music makes me want to dance!

"OUT" OF YOUR BODY

*I'm sluggish.
I need a cup of coffee.*

*I need stronger drugs
for my backache.*

*I'm too fat
to go to the gym.*

*I need to step
outside for a smoke.*

*That bag of cookies was gone
before I knew it!*

*I had a rough day—
I'm skipping dinner and going
straight for dessert.*

*Dancing makes
me look foolish.*

A healthy relationship with your body is the sum of many individual decisions you make every day.

the times of day that work best for both of you can make the difference between frustration and fireworks.

Fun Ways of Getting Back in Your Body

Besides training yourself to be more conscious of factors relating to your body's needs, there are any number of recreational activities that will automatically help you get back in your body. They may sound simple, and they are! But don't discount what they have to offer. Here are just a few:

➤ **Learn how to *play*.** If that requires explanation, seek out the experts: Spend more time with kids and animals and let them show you how it's done!

➤ **Tackle a new physical skill.** Whether it's fencing, singing, or sailing, mastering a new skill teaches you about your body, promotes self-esteem, and enlarges your world.

➤ **Cultivate sensory awareness.** Becoming more alive to your senses is certainly one of the best parts of being in your body. A way to do this is to approach sensory experience in a conscious, meditative frame of mind. The next chapter will explain how.

➤ **Take Body Appreciation 101.** Find ways to explore your body through knowledge. Learn more about its systems and stages of life. Do this through reading and talking with older friends. For extra credit, sign up for an anatomy class at your local community college.

➤ **Explore the arts and music.** There's hardly an aspect of music or art that doesn't bring you more into your body. Throwing pots, painting, playing an instrument—all require developing your physical skills and are rich with sensory payoff.

➤ **Grow and cook your own food.** The whole cycle of food— from the labor of tending a vegetable garden to the pleasure of filling the house with mouthwatering aromas—involves your body in a primal, sensual experience. Not to mention that food can be extremely sexy!

> **Give a massage.** Receiving a massage can feel wonderful, but learning to *give* a massage is a real education in the human body, and can be a great exercise in body awareness. (I'll cover some favorite self-massage techniques in the next chapter.)

My Five Body-Awareness Questions to Ask . . .

Wherever you go, whatever you do, your body is along for the ride. Don't neglect it. Here are five quick check-in questions to pose in various situations. You might feel like Jiminy Cricket asking yourself these questions, but you'll go a long way toward keeping the mind–body relationship intact and healthy.

On a Night Out

1. If I'm drinking alcohol, am I drinking sufficient water to help my body process it?

   Drink at least one large glass of water after any alcoholic beverage.

2. Is the music louder than I can comfortably talk over?

   If so, you might be permanently damaging your ears. Buy some plastic or foam earplugs, or, in a pinch, roll up a cocktail napkin into a tight plug and stuff your ears (leaving enough to easily pull out).

3. Am I breathing smoke, and, if so, how can I avoid it?

4. Did I bring a sweater or jacket so I don't catch cold?

5. Am I pushing myself to party beyond my desire or energy to do so?

At the Table

1. Am I experiencing a craving, or genuine hunger?

2. Is my hunger connected to an uncomfortable feeling or situation?

3. Am I eating automatically, or am I really tasting the food?

4. Am I eating a good balance of nutrients?

5. Am I remembering to eat slowly enough to allow the feeling of satiety to catch up with me?

At the Gym

1. How's my energy level; do I need a quick energy snack before starting?

2. Am I focused on what I'm doing or is my mind wandering to what I'm going to do later in the day?

3. Am I working in the range that fits my goals? Am I making the right adjustments to my pace, my form, and my weights, in order to keep working at the level I want?

   If you're recovering from injury, are you working too hard? If you're working to build muscle, are you working out hard enough? If you're prone to over-doing it, are you pacing yourself?

4. Am I tuned into my progress?

   Look at what you can do that you couldn't do before. Feel for the burn. Enjoy the sensation of breathing well, of developing power. Try to feel, in the moment, what you're getting out of it.

5. Am I carefully monitoring myself to distinguish "good" pain (the heat of the muscular effort) from "bad" pain (the sharp pain of injury)?

With Your Kids

1. Am I lifting them without strain to my back?

   To pick up a child from the floor, bend at your knees—not at your waist. Squat down, tighten your stomach muscles, and lift with your legs. To place a child in a car seat, kneel on the backseat while you lift the child into the seat.

2. Am I always carrying them on the same hip or shoulder?

3. Am I fixing food for myself, or always just picking at their plates?

4. When was the last time I looked in the mirror, got dressed, showered, or took care of any personal hygiene?

5. Am I taking advantage of their downtime to get my physical needs met?

Making Love

1. Does the anticipation of sexual activity produce feelings of pleasure and excitement? If not, why not?

2. Am I aroused, and am I comfortable being aroused? What alternatives do we have if I don't feel aroused, or would rather not be right now?

3. Am I present and able to focus on this experience?

4. Is there any possibility of sexually transmitted disease, and have I protected myself appropriately?

5. (Afterward) Does sex itself produce a feeling of satisfaction, relaxation, and enjoyment? If not, why not?

In the Car

1. Is my sitting posture producing tension anywhere in my body, and can I adjust myself to reduce the tension?

2. How long have I been driving without a break?

3. Am I eating in the car?

4. Am I delaying physical needs—to use the bathroom, to eat, to stretch—which might cause my body distress?

5. Am I feeling drowsy?

   If so, don't risk any other remedies such as playing the radio—immediately stop and take a nap!

Traveling

1. Am I making sure I'm well rested *before* I go?

2. If I'm flying, am I drinking a pint of water for every hour in the air?

3. How can I keep some semblance of my exercise program going? Does my hotel have a fitness facility?

4. If the trip will last less than three days, can I stay on my home time?

    This will help minimize jet lag on short trips.

5. (For a trip of more than three days) Once at my destination, am I keeping up a regular schedule of eating, exercise, and sleep, adjusted to local time?

    This will speed the adjustment to local time on longer trips.

At the End of the Day

1. Do I feel good about my food and exercise today?

2. Did I allow any quiet time to relax, to meditate, to think, to recharge?

3. Did I stress my body unnecessarily?

4. Am I relaxed enough to fall asleep, or should I do some stretching, or take a hot bath?

5. Am I setting myself up for a good day tomorrow?

Exercise: Living in the Moment

Imagine you've come to one of those crossroads in the day when you're not sure exactly what to do with yourself. *I should go for a walk. I should eat something. I should clean the house.* Stop the "shoulds" for a moment. Try listening to your body without imposing any ideas on it. Sit and listen: What physical urges are being held at bay in your body? For example, what sounds would come out if you let them? You might be surprised. Would you scream? Would you roar? Try breathing a couple of big sighs, using your voice. Let each one become longer and freer, until you feel the sounds are coming from the deepest part of you. Don't judge what you're doing or how it sounds—simply let it out.

Now sit quietly and feel your weight in your muscles and limbs. What position would your body assume if you let it? Would you flop on the ground? Would you curl up in a ball? Would you jump up and down? Maybe your eyes would close if you didn't hold them open. Maybe you'd feel like turning off the lights and sitting in the dark. Maybe you'd climb into a cool bath, or just take off all your clothes and dance in front of the mirror, pretending to be a rock star. Why not go with it? Let your body express what it wants to express. Try this once a day, until you find yourself responding to situations more spontaneously *without* having to tell yourself to.

When it comes to living in the body, the need to honor the body's cycles exists side by side with the imperative to honor the moment. After all, spontaneity is where the fun, the richness, the intensity of life come from. Having a healthy routine in place is important, but equally important are those sudden poetic impulses that make you unique. If that means a detour from routine, fine. There are mornings to skip the gym and sleep in late with your husband. There are chocolate cakes too good to pass up. Give yourself the freedom to live in the moment. Some days, the routine can wait—because life won't.

CHAPTER 6

Sense and Sensuality

Developing Greater Sensory Awareness

Flex Appeal Is: ✔ *Expanding your capacity for pleasure.*

HOW DO YOU THINK about your *sensuality?* What does it have to do with your *senses?* And how does sensuality relate to sexuality? These are the sorts of questions I've been asking women lately.

Words like *sensory, sensual, sensuous,* and *sexual* often run together. Of course, though, each means something slightly different.

Back in the days of petticoats and top hats, *sensuous* was the polite term—it meant the type of aesthetic pleasure you got from things like music, art, and nature. *Sensual* meant carnal, sexual. Today, these two terms get used interchangeably and, to many, have simply become other words for "sex." But most women I talk with see an important distinction between their sensuality and their sexuality.

Sensuality Versus Sexuality

Many sensual experiences are pleasurable without being sexual. As one of my readers wrote: "Wearing a fuzzy sweater on a chilly day, hugging my sons, hearing my partner's voice, and eating runny Camembert cheese are some of the sensual highlights of my life." Sensuality is a quality, an awareness, a way of living. Not everyone places the same value on it. But, for many of us, sensuality and passion are closely related.

One woman told me, "I don't like to be called 'sexy,' but when a man says, 'Oh, she's so *sensual*,' it makes me think he sees more than just the equipment—that he sees deeper into the soul." She went on to say that being appreciated as a *sensual* being, rather than a *sexual* one, helps her feel more complete—ultimately freeing her to be more open physically and sexually.

For many of us, sensuality is the fuse leading to sexual passion. And *sensory* pleasures are the match that lights the fuse.

Sensory experience → Sensuality → Sexuality

Still, getting in touch with the pleasures of our senses is not always easy to do—partly because that quiet era of petticoats and top hats is long gone.

Sensory Overload

Every day, we surf a tidal wave of stimulation—of noise and imagery, fast travel and global communication. Stimulation, though, is not the same as sensation. In fact, constant stimulation *deadens* sensation. It's as though you rubbed the same patch of skin on your arm over and over: First, it would stop feeling good, then it would stop feeling at all. Finally, it would be rubbed raw.

Sensuality is something completely different from the daily sensory

Listening to my favorite music, working out, exploring nature —
all these things enhance my sensuality.

—Luanne, thirty-nine, Aurora, Indiana

overdose we get from pop culture and technology. Sensuality is a reaching-out to explore and experience the subtle pleasures of the natural world.

In the same way that New York City would be unthinkable without the sprawling green sanctuary of Central Park at its heart, life in modern society would be impossible to bear without a connection to nature, to quiet, and to subtlety.

In this chapter, we'll discuss ways of expanding sensory awareness as a prelude to greater sensuality.

Sensory Awareness Meditation

How does someone practice sensory awareness?

To practice sensing, you meditate on the *process* of your senses. That is, you mindfully tune into the experience of your senses.

Think back to the first time you experienced some particularly wonderful sensation. It could be your first kiss, your first snowfall, or the first time you smelled your baby's skin. Those "firsts" remain vivid because their newness held you, kept you present, during the experience.

Sensory awareness meditation is our means of re-creating that first-time freshness.

Barring some abnormality, all of us have sensory organs that are working all the time. The question is whether we're having a rich sensory experience, or only a superficial one. A rich sensory experience demands two things: *slowing down* and *mindful awareness.*

Step 1. Slowing Down

Things naturally become more sensual if you slow them down. The simple act of washing your hands can be anything from a perfunctory splash-and-rinse to a luxurious ritual, depending on how fast or slow you do it. This is because, for an act to become sensual, you literally need to allow *time* for the processing of sensations. Take something as automatic as picking up a pencil to write. Do it slowly, giving your senses time to explore its color, weight, temperature, and texture—and this simple act becomes fascinating.

When I began exploring sensual dance movements, my body quickly taught me the connection between slowness and sensuality. I found that slowing the tempo gave my body a chance to "feel" into the move—that is, to really sink into it physically and emotionally.

Step 2. Mindful Awareness

Once you've slowed down, you're not only open to sensation; unfortunately, you're also open to distractions. All sorts of random thoughts and anxieties can flood in to fill the time: *This is silly. I feel stupid. What's for dinner?* That's why sensory awareness also requires *mindfulness.* You have to give that time over to your senses. This means keeping your awareness focused. Move at the body's own pace and rhythm, and allow your senses to engage for as long as they are intrigued.

If you do this, it's likely that your senses will draw you deeper and deeper into the discovery of savory minutiae.

EXERCISE: MINDFUL MOMENTS

As you go through your day, occasionally choose a task and carry it out in a slower, more deliberate, and receptive state. Do this with tasks that are normally unconscious: putting on socks and shoes, using your door key, washing your hands. See how it feels to perform these tasks at an extremely slow speed; spend half a minute picking up your coffee cup and taking a sip, and so on. It may feel very strange—as though you're drugged or sleepwalking. Notice how easy it is to become distracted by outside thoughts, and how tough it is to maintain your concentration on the sensory experience. As you notice your mind wandering, direct it back to your sensations.

The Benefits of Mindful Sensory Awareness

Although I've been talking about the process of consciously engaging your senses, that's not to say the senses don't engage *unconsciously* all the time—

all of us are grabbed by things. We look up and gasp at a sunset, or melt into a back rub, or smell a pie baking. These are hard to miss.

But there's a world of subtler sensation that often goes unnoticed. And it's these subtleties that you'll discover through mindful awareness—in the same way that you spot more stars as your eyes adjust to the darkness. In fact, even those high-voltage sensations—those sunsets and brass bands—become richer, more exciting, more nuanced, when you experience them consciously. That is, when you focus consciously on the physical thrill they're causing.

If you don't believe conscious attention and pleasure are connected, try kissing your partner while balancing on one foot. You might succeed, but it probably won't be the best kiss you ever enjoyed. The more conscious, undivided attention we give to our senses, the richer the experience will be.

The benefits of conscious, mindful sensory awareness are:

> Our senses become more acute.

> We gain more information about the world around us.

> We perceive more accurately.

> We learn to live in the moment.

> We experience more pleasure from the things we perceive.

In the next section, I'll offer a number of sensory exercises for you to have fun with. Here are two tips for engaging in mindful sensory awareness:

> **Isolate your senses.** We rely so much on our eyes that we easily overlook data coming in through other channels. When someone sneaks up behind you, puts her hands over your eyes, and says, "Guess who!" you know her instantly by her touch, her voice, and perhaps her scent. Guess what? That same data is all there when you meet her face to face, but once your eyes have identified her, you don't consciously register the other information. In the exercises that follow, I've isolated the senses to heighten the experience.

➤ **Jump in without** *thinking.* Our senses operate nonverbally. Your exploration will be richer if you can experience things directly and intimately without thinking *about* them. Try to focus on the physical experience—the sound, color, or taste—rather than on the label you might attach to it. Rather than saying to yourself *I hear a bird chirping,* focus on the abstract qualities of the sound—its rhythm, its range, and its tonality. Imagine how the experience of saying *It's a swimming pool* would compare with simply jumping in!

Sensory 2 Exercises

If you wanted to, you could simply declare a "sensory awareness day" and spend it soaking up as much sensory stimulation as possible, without labeling it or responding to it with thoughts. As an alternative, however, this section contains specific exercises for isolated senses. Think of them as games, and enjoy playing them! When you've tried these, create some of your own.

Thanks to writer and Jungian therapist James Harvey Stout, now deceased, for some of the exercises that follow, adapted from his self-published work *The Human Handbook,* which is now available as *The Human LifeBook: A Lucid Guide to Conscious Living in the New Millennium.*

Seeing

Sight is generally our dominant sense. Yet much passes before our eyes that we don't savor. Here are two very different sight awareness exercises: one designed to enhance mindfulness, the other to teach awareness through deprivation.

A VISUAL DIARY

There's no better way to really see something than to draw it. Don't worry if you're not an artist. You don't have to show this to anyone. Carry a small sketchbook with you and, when you find yourself with fifteen or thirty minutes to spare, sit and draw whatever you see. It doesn't matter if it's a park fountain or the waiting room in the dentist's office. Pick a detail of the scene—a cup, a chair, a leaf—and study it line by line, angle by angle. You'll find that objects you draw may remain in your mind for years to come.

FLATTENING THE WORLD

Because sight is our most used sense, it can be very interesting to go without it for a period of time. In this exercise, you'll change your visual experience by removing your sense of depth perception. Cover one eye with a patch or scarf and spend twenty minutes exploring the world two-dimensionally. (Don't try to drive while doing this, and be very careful walking so you don't bump into walls or furniture!) Experiment performing simple tasks: Try tossing a ball into the air and catching it. Try picking up things and setting them down. Notice what other visual cues you begin to rely on in order to navigate three-dimensionally. Reach out your hand to an object. Does the size of the object help you estimate its distance? Notice how things in the foreground seem to move faster than things in the background. After twenty minutes, remove the patch. Does your sense of depth seem heightened? Spend some time meditating on your renewed awareness of three-dimensional reality.

Hearing

AMBIENT AWARENESS

Close your eyes and listen to the sounds around you for ten minutes. Depending on where you are, you may hear traffic, voices, the hum of a refrigerator, birds, sirens, rain, or a hundred other things. Imagine yourself floating around, above, and through the sounds you hear. Don't label any of it as noise; imagine that what you are hearing is music, and every sound is a new phrase. Try this in the bathtub, on a park bench, in a library, or anywhere else you think of.

ACCIDENTAL SOUND

Begin some chore or task—perhaps sweeping or cleaning, gardening or working at your desk—and listen closely to each sound that is created.

CAN YOU HEAR ME NOW?

In a quiet room, turn on a radio to a very low volume so that you have to listen intently to hear it. As a variation, play the radio at normal volume, but then slowly move away from it, and try to continue to hear it from ever-increasing distances.

LISTENING TO YOUR BODY

Put a finger gently into each ear, and listen to the sounds within your body. Listen for your breathing, your heartbeat, your swallowing. Listen to the sounds of your vertebrae as you move your head from side to side. Hum a long tone, and listen to your own voice coming to you through the bones of your skull.

MUSICAL ISOLATION EXERCISE

Here's an ear training exercise given to me by a musician: Listen to a song or classical piece and focus on a single instrument (not the voice). Try to screen out the other parts of the music and follow *only* what that one instrument is playing.

RESONANCE MEDITATION

Get a bell, finger cymbal, metal chime, or any metallic piece that rings when you strike it. Hit it and listen carefully to the fading of the sound.

Smelling

SMELL SWATCHES

Create an aromatic extravaganza for your nose—a buffet of fragrances: flowers of various kinds, incense, soap, cedar chips, pipe tobacco, perfume or cologne, or foods and spices from your kitchen. Systematically investigate each of them, noting its character.

SENSE MEMORY

As you smell a fragrance, notice whether it triggers a specific memory, and whether it changes your mood or your state.

FOLLOWING YOUR NOSE

Walk throughout your home or backyard with eyes closed. (Be careful not to stumble.) Notice the subtle odors from room to room, from house to yard.

NOSE TEASE

Select something with an aroma that you find especially tantalizing—a few drops of your husband's cologne, a gardenia, what have you—and place it several feet away from you while you read or work. Put it just out of smell's reach, so that only the slightest hint of it will drift into your awareness every few minutes.

Tasting

KITCHEN SAFARI

The taste buds in your mouth detect four main categories of tastes: sweet, bitter, sour, and salty. In order to detect the true flavor of a food—the difference between an apple and a pear—you also rely on signals from olfactory receptors in the nose and soft palate, as well as the distinctive consistency of the food in your mouth. Explore your kitchen, sampling different foods, and try to categorize each one according to its predominant quality of sweet, bitter, sour, or salty. You can try holding your nose to help you isolate the taste. Try an olive, a bite of cheese, a bit of dried fruit, some chocolate, a few coffee grounds, a walnut, and so on. Once you've categorized them, try different combinations of two qualities. Put a drop of honey on top of an almond and taste the result. Try other combinations as the inspiration strikes you.

THE SPICE RACK

Taste a pinch of each of the spices in your kitchen. (I suggest rinsing your mouth between tastes.)

BLIND WINE TASTING

This one's fun with a group. Buy three different bottles of wine and serve tastes from plain brown wrappers. Compare each wine to professional tasters' descriptions your wine merchant can supply you with. You and your guests try to match the samples with the correct descriptions. Then pull off the wrappers and see how you did. Alternatively, you can try this idea with nonalcoholic gourmet items, including coffees, green teas, cheeses, or chocolates.

EXPLORE LIKE A BABY

Put various objects into your mouth to taste them. Objects might include a pen, a key, a crystal, a quarter, your thumb, and so on. (Be sure to "childproof" your items by washing them first, and don't use anything poisonous!)

LIFESAVER GAME

Open a package of LifeSavers or another candy that comes in multiple flavors. Without looking at it, place a candy in your mouth and *hold your nostrils shut* while you try to guess the flavor. Try again with other colors.

DON'T SPIT IT OUT (THIS TIME)

Taste a food you don't like. (Liver, anyone? Coffee? Anchovies? Lima beans?) Withhold judgment; instead, try to enter completely into the taste on its own terms and experience its true character as an impartial observer.

Touch

TEXTURE SWATCHES

Collect a variety of fabrics and materials. These might include velvet, nylon, fur, wood, steel, plastic, clay, and others. Select items with different tactile qualities: smooth, rough, wet, slimy. Now touch each one, as though each held a secret that you could feel with your fingers. Keep them in a box and sort through them occasionally with eyes closed.

FEELING AT HOME

Walk through your home, slowly, mindfully touching the furniture and other articles. Seek out a variety of textures and qualities.

HOT 'N' COLD DANCE

Hold a mug containing a hot beverage in one hand and a glass of ice water in the other. Close your eyes and focus on the simultaneous experience of hot and cold. After about a minute, cross your arms and hold each hand up to the opposite side of your face, pressing the mug and glass against your cheeks. Hold the liquids against your face with your eyes closed for another minute, again feeling the signals of hot and cold circling through your nervous system. Finally, switch both liquids to the opposite hands and notice what happens to your perception.

THIS IS ME

Touch your skin on various parts of your body, and notice both the sensation received from the hand that's touching, as well as the spot being touched. Be aware of such qualities as texture, temperature, oiliness, hairiness, and tone. Touch yourself in various ways—tickling, scratching, rubbing, tapping, or stroking. *Extra-Sensual Variation:* Explore the skin of your partner.

BLIND DRAWING

Draw your partner's face without looking at it, by exploring it with your free hand as you draw. You can also do this with an object.

SWEET DREAMS

Your mother probably taught you to sleep in a T-shirt in case there's a fire. But take a chance: Try sleeping *au naturel* and enjoy the sensation of crisp, clean sheets against bare skin all night long.

NO FINGERPRINTS

Instead of touching objects only with your hands, touch them with other parts of your body—your forearms, bare feet, or head.

PARTNER EXERCISE

Explore your partner's body with your bare feet.

This is one of my favorites. Close your eyes and explore your partner's body with one hand while simultaneously mirroring your movements on your own body with the other hand. Make sure you touch the identical spots with each hand. As your hands map the terrain of your bodies, let the maps overlay each other in your mind's eye. Begin with nonintimate areas, and progress only as you're both comfortable. This exercise can create a feeling of intimacy even beyond the sensory experience.

My Ten-Minute Refreshingly Sensual Self-Massage with Oil

No exploration of the senses would be complete without including the sensory delights of massage. Gentle massage is soothing and healing; yet although we instinctively rub a bumped shin or tired eyelids, most of us don't often treat ourselves to more extensive self-massage. This simple oil massage is adapted from ayurvedic tradition.

Self-Massage with Oil

Oil massage is considered a preventive in ayurvedic medicine. It is designed to tone the skin, smooth out the muscles, stimulate circulation of blood and lymph, and leave your body feeling wonderfully sleek and alive. Sesame seed oil, olive oil, canola oil, almond oil, or coconut oil may be used. If you're buying a prepared massage oil, make sure it has one of these oils as the main ingredient. When I have time, I like to blend sesame and almond oil and add a bit of essential oil such as frankincense, lavender, or eucalyptus for a "scent"-sational massage. On a hot summer day, coconut oil is wonderful.

This massage is usually done standing up, and should be done naked. For best results, leave the oil on your body for at least ninety minutes before showering off. I like to do this massage just after a shower in the evening. I towel off the excess oil, put on my comfortable nightclothes, and enjoy the lingering sensations before going to bed. The oil is completely absorbed by the time I climb into the sheets.

Oil Massage Technique

Unlike in Swedish massage, the hands do not knead or dig deeply into the muscles. Instead, the palms remain flat and are brushed, or drawn, evenly over the skin with only moderate pressure, as though you were smoothing wrinkles from a bedsheet.

In the ayurvedic tradition, oil massage is often done at a brisk tempo that can actually be aerobic if done for thirty minutes or more. But I like to do it at a slow, steady pace that allows time to enjoy the sensations. Feel free to linger over an area for greater stimulation. Try spending extra time on your ankles, wrists, backs of the knees, or any area that feels especially good.

Take your time to master the movements, making sure to cover your whole body with oil.

1. Place a few drops of oil in your palm and rub the hands together. You will add oil as needed, but will require less and less oil the more often you do this massage.

2. Begin by rubbing the tips of the fingers, then move through your body in the sequence below:

FACE AND HEAD

1. Rub the top of your head in a circular motion, then massage upward from the hairline to the top of the head—*all the way around the head*.

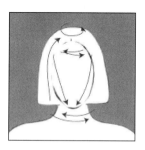

2. Rub across your forehead in both directions. Rub downward along the sides of your face from your temples across your cheekbones, across the chin and upper lip, and along the sides of the nose.

3. Rub the right palm across the front of the throat moving from left to right, then switch hands and move from right to left. Alternate back and forth.

SHOULDERS AND BACK OF HEAD

4. Rub the back of your neck by crossing your left palm over the right side of the neck and drawing it clear around to the front, then crossing your right palm over your left shoulder and drawing it similarly around front. Alternate hands.

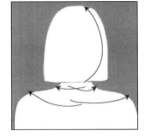

5. Rub from the nape of the neck to the crown of the head.

FRONT TORSO

6. Rub your stomach in a circular motion clockwise, then counter-clockwise. Start at the navel and make bigger circles as you go. Complete about one circle per second. The goal is to completely cover the area with oil, so you can continue as long as it feels good.

7. Rub across the chest with long diagonal strokes. Begin by lifting the right arm up over your head. Then, use your left hand to stroke from the underside of the right arm, over the armpit, and above the breast to the sternum. Make a second stroke from the inner arm, across the armpit, to just *under* the breast. Alternate these two strokes, then switch sides and repeat.

ARMS, LEGS, BUTTOCKS, AND SIDES

8. Using long strokes, rub along the long bones of your body (arms and legs). Move downward from the shoulder and armpit to the fingertips, rotating the arm at the shoulder so you rub both front

and back of each arm. Then finally, use a series of wringing motions, lightly squeezing and twisting the flesh back and forth along the entire length of the arm from wrist to armpit, and the leg from ankles to upper inner thighs.

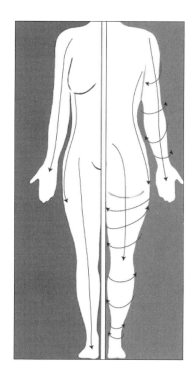

9. Rub the whole side of the body from the armpit to the thigh in long downward strokes. Alternate sides.

10. Using long downward strokes, reach back and rub the buttocks— alternate left and right side from the small of the back over the buttocks to the thighs. Alternate back and forth.

FEET

11. Finally, massage across the tops of your feet. Rub the back of the heels and the arches. Rub your toes.

PART III

The Program

CHAPTER 7

Flex Appeal Basics

I'VE DONE LOTS of photo sessions, but the shoot for this book was one of the longest ever!

Typically, to capture an exercise on film, I may spend two or three minutes—sometimes more—holding a position that may account for only thirty seconds in the final routine. This means that, by the end of the day, I've done all the routines in the book three or four times each.

And so, given how many exercises there are in this program, I was prepared for a marathon. What I *wasn't* prepared for was how good it would feel.

As I worked through each section of my body in front of the camera, I was amazed at how the exercises would highlight areas of tension, and then release them. I'd start a neck stretch and realize I'd been walking around for days not knowing how tense I was there. Then, after a few minutes, that area would be feeling supple and energized. I'd move to a new area, spotlight the tension there, and release. It was like moving through my body with an oil can.

The next day, instead of feeling wiped out, my body felt amazing—I felt revitalized.

Sweating the Small Things

This experience helped confirm the unique benefits of *Flex Appeal*. It's not about athletic performance, or climbing mountains—that type of all-out activity is fun, too, but this is something different. *Flex Appeal* is about working through the day-to-day tensions and stiffness—the subtle annoyances that prevent you from participating in life. It's also about strengthening and toning muscle to help you live with greater vitality.

Whenever you're tired, stiff, or just not feeling great, you can get into one of the program's restful, grounding poses and feel the tension and fatigue melting away. Likewise, when you're stressed, you can use the more invigorating poses to blast that pent-up energy right *through* your body—purging yourself emotionally and recharging your batteries.

In this way, *Flex Appeal* does what I said in the first chapter: opens your body to new possibilities—both physically and emotionally. When some part of your body doesn't feel right, it takes attention away from enjoyment. *Flex Appeal* brings back the possibility of enjoying your body.

Sensual Movement Basics

In preparation for starting our workout, let's look at some of the special characteristics of the *Flex Appeal* routines. First, I'll discuss two of the most important principles: the *fluid body* and the *breath*. Then I'll talk about the qualities and patterns of movements you'll be doing.

The Fluid Body

As I described in chapter 2, everything in *Flex Appeal* is aimed at strengthening, toning, and limbering, all in the context of becoming more *fluid*. If that sounds a little abstract and you're wondering what it really means, let me try to instill in your mind a set of images to guide you in these exercises. It's the imagery of what I call the fluid body.

Try to imagine your body in liquid terms, as opposed to solid. In reality, our bodies are 70 percent water—even our solid tissues are mostly water. But the *fluid body* refers not only to the actual fluids in the body—the blood, lymph, synovial fluid, spinal fluids, and water—but also to the variety of integrated, fluid *movements* made possible as you gain more flexibility and freedom in your joints. In addition, it refers to the fluid circulation of *energy* that drives these movements. As you move various parts of your body in the exercises, it may help you to visualize waves, ripples, or pouring streams of liquid. Little by little you'll find yourself translating the metaphor into motion.

The Breath

If you were to search for the life force in your body—if you wanted *proof* of life—it would be your breath. You can breathe hard, as you do when you're exercising, or quietly as when you sleep; you can breathe consciously or unconsciously, but your breath is a rhythm that never stops.

In a physical sense, the breath delivers oxygen, our body's most constant requirement. But in psychic terms, breath also is a conduit of emotions, of sexual vitality—of everything that we call *spirit*. In addition to keeping us alive and vital, the breath creates a connection between our outer environment and our inner self.

Breathing is integral to the movement in these routines. As you become more adept at the exercises, breath and movement should become intertwined in such a way that stretching leads you to breathe, and breathing leads you to stretch.

UJJAYI BREATHING

The style of breath we'll use in these exercises is called *ujjayi* (oo-JAI-ee) breathing. Ujjayi breathing is produced by softly whispering the long syllable *ahhhh*—as you let your breath out and in, slowly and evenly. The slight pressure at the back of the palate makes the breathing audible, like the hush of the ocean in a cave, and regulates the speed of the air, helping keep the tempo smooth and slow. When you are performing the exercises, ujjayi breathing should be done with your mouth closed.

BREATH OF FIRE (KAPALABHATI)

Several of the exercises call for a special type of breathing known as Breath of Fire. This rapid nasal breathing "fires" you up and stimulates metabolic processes. Breathing only through the nose, pull your navel toward your lower back to create the exhale. Then soften your belly and let the inhale come naturally. Pulse the exhales rapidly, relaxing between each exhale to let the air flow back in.

Women with an IUD should not do Breath of Fire.

PLACEMENT OF THE BREATH

Typically, in resistance exercise, the part of a movement requiring the most exertion is done on the exhale. As you move through the postures in *Flex Appeal,* however, other principles will also apply at times:

➤ Whenever your body is folding or closing, compacting in on itself, the movement should be accompanied by an *exhale.*

➤ When your body is twisting, *exhale* to let the air out and facilitate the twist.

➤ When you are releasing your body to the pull of gravity, *exhale* to facilitate the stretch.

➤ When your body is opening, unfolding, or straightening in some way, the movement should be done on an *inhale.*

➤ During a held pose where you are expanding your spine, the *inhale* expands the spine, while the *exhale* grounds and stabilizes the spine's expansion.

In many of the exercises, I have indicated *inhale* and *exhale* to help you find the correct rhythm. If, after experimenting, you find other ways to integrate the breath with the movement that feel more natural to you, feel free to follow your body's lead.

Movement Focus

The exercises are designed to evoke a variety of responses in the body. They span a range of energies from restful grounding poses, through movements designed to awaken or warm up your body, to movements meant to energize, or really work, the muscles and joints. There are also rejuvenating poses to help you cool down and bring your awareness inward. Along the way, I've provided descriptions or bits of imagery to help you discover or vary the qualities of the movements you're doing.

Sensual Movement

Central to this program, of course, is the special quality of sensual movement.

Unlike the more goal-oriented and externally driven movements in most fitness programs, sensual movements are internally driven—sparked by the creative, playful spirit within you.

Sensual energy is created by doing the movements:

➤ Slowly

➤ Smoothly

➤ With mindful emphasis on the parts of your body that are moving

The fun part is that you don't have to think to yourself: *I am now going to be sensual.* If you do any movement—if you rotate your hips, for instance—following all three of these guidelines, I guarantee that your brain will get the message your body is sending!

As you move through these routines, simply concentrate on going with the flow. Follow what feels good. Gradually, you will begin to trust the inner flow of movement within you.

Sensual Movement Patterns

Sensual movement patterns are the vehicle that allow the body to "flow"—to move to its own rhythm and current. These movements create harmony and vitality by uniting the rhythms of body and breath. They have other benefits as well—for example, alleviating menstrual and menopausal distresses by improving the flow of energy in the pelvic region. Plus, they greatly increase the power of the poses to tone and strengthen the muscles.

Here's a preview of some of the types of movement you'll be doing while in these poses.

CIRCLE

The circle is the most basic pattern in these exercises. Many body parts will move through a circle, including your arms, hips, legs, and torso. Circles create a continuum of movement that improves circulation in your joints and induces deep states of relaxation and meditation.

WAVE

The wave is a motion in which a curve moves *through* your body—usually along your spine—in much the same way a wave ripples through water. When you perform a wave, the goal is to "find" as many joints in the chain as you can and let the energy move through each of them in turn.

SEMICIRCLE

A semicircle is an arc or pendulum movement, used in some exercises to begin warming up your joints to do full circles.

TWIST

The twist is a wringing movement of your spine.

PREPARATION FOR BELLY DANCE OR OTHER SENSUAL DANCE FORMS

If you're interested in further exploring the aesthetic and sensual nature of these exercises, I encourage you to experiment with other dance forms as you progress. If you do, you'll find the *Flex Appeal* routines are ideal preparation. Middle Eastern dance (or belly dancing), for instance, offers you a way to build flexibility and strength while participating in an art form that started more than two thousand years ago. Originally a spiritual celebration of the feminine power of fertility and childbearing, it's now a fun and sensual way to take your *Flex Appeal* training to another level.

Circles done while a body part is also moving linearly through space produce a spiral pattern. An example would be circling your hips while bending your knees.

FIGURE-8

Figure-8s stimulate sensual flow in your hips and wrists. They are created by alternating circles with your hips, or with alternating over- and underhanded circles with your wrists. Like circles, the continuous movement of figure-8s creates a relaxing and meditative state while increasing circulation in your joints.

General Guidelines for Doing the *Flex Appeal* Routines

Safety

All these moves, if done gently and slowly, will help loosen and lengthen the muscles, reducing tension and lubricating joints. They are designed to be therapeutic, but can be stressful if done too quickly or forcefully. You should check with your doctor before beginning this or any exercise program, especially if you have any preexisting back, neck, or shoulder injury.

Here are some general safety rules:

➤ **Keep movements small while you're learning them.** They can become bigger and more free as you gain confidence.

➤ **Don't jerk or force the moves.**

➤ **Go slowly, especially when warming up.**

➤ **Be sensitive to variations in tightness in your body, and don't overstress the limber areas.** You might find, for example, that your hips are naturally looser than your middle back. If so, concentrate on using the movement to gently loosen up the areas that are most rigid, rather than excessively working the parts that already move freely.

> ➤ Stop if you feel pain or pinching in joints.
> ➤ Spinal Twists are not advisable for women who are pregnant.

Of course, always check with your doctor if you have any concerns about whether these exercises are appropriate for you.

Time and Rep Guidelines

The duration of most exercises is given in seconds (for a held pose), or in repetitions of a movement, called reps. In a few cases, the duration is given in breaths, in which case your breathing will provide the length and/or the count for the exercise.

These time and rep guidelines are suggestions. Think of them as goals, and work toward them over time. Don't push yourself beyond your comfort zone at first.

Modifications

For some of the exercises, I've included modifiers to help you make the exercise easier or harder as needed. As you become stronger and more fluid, you can also use tempo as a means of increasing the challenge. These exercises will actually become aerobic if you move steadily through them at a fast tempo. Once again, though, don't speed up the movements until your body is comfortable doing them slowly.

Dances

You'll notice that some of the exercises have the word *dance* as part of their name. This is an invitation to let your body move as fluidly and sensually as you can. In the dances, try to go beyond the letter of the movement and enter into the spirit by allowing yourself to improvise and go with the flow of your own inspiration. In short, let go and have fun!

Music

Everyone knows the old adage of a picture being worth a thousand words. In the case of dance and movement, the right *music* is worth a thousand words—and pictures, too, for that matter—in teaching your body what to do. I find that my body always performs in a more fluid, intuitive way when there's music playing. Slow, rhythmic, sensual music works best. It could be anything from slow blues to Sade (my personal favorite), Middle Eastern dance music, or whatever else makes your body feel loose and sexy. Choose music that gets *you* in the mood. See Resources and Recommended Reading for more suggestions.

Glossary

Some of the words in these descriptions may seem strange, especially if you've never been exposed to yoga poses. Following is a short glossary of some potentially unfamiliar terms.

- ➤ **Feel into** means to bring your attention to a physical area or sensation.

- ➤ **Root** means to visualize a solid foundation or connection to the Earth, as in *root your feet down*.

- ➤ The **pubic bone** is the ridge of bone in the center of your groin.

- ➤ To **soften** a muscle means to consciously relax it. For example, you might be instructed to soften your neck muscles during an exercise in which you are stretching your arms, and where the natural tendency would be to tense the neck as well.

- ➤ To **release** means to relax and allow a stretch to occur.

- ➤ The **sitbones** are the ischial tuberosities—the two bony knobs on the underside of your pelvis that you sit on.

- ➤ The **sacrum** is a triangular plate of bone composed of five fused vertebrae at the base of the spine.

➤ **Firm around the sitbones** means to contract your glutes and hamstrings; in other words, tense your buttocks.

➤ To **stack** the hips or knees means to line them up, one over the other.

How to Approach the Routines

The next four chapters are self-contained routines for four areas of the body. I recommend sticking with these basic routines until you've learned the exercises:

➤ Chapter 8: Core and Spine

➤ Chapter 9: Hips, Pelvis, and Legs

➤ Chapter 10: Upper Body

➤ Chapter 11: Face and Head

Although these are complete, sequenced routines, it's not essential to go through an entire routine on a given day—nevertheless, let that be your goal.

Once you've mastered the basic routines, you can begin to explore the extra routines provided in chapter 12. These specialized routines use exercises from the four basic routines, resequenced to emphasize a particular quality or goal:

➤ Special Routine 1: Fluid Relaxation Meditation

➤ Special Routine 2: Sensual Strength and Weight Loss

➤ Special Routine 3: *Flex Appeal* Dance

A Note on Learning the Exercises

There are a lot of exercises in this program, each with detailed instructions. While this may seem daunting at first, you'll find that your body will learn these exercises after only a few workouts.

CREATE YOUR OWN INSTRUCTION TAPE

To help yourself learn the exercises, one method is to read the instructions into a tape recorder. This will save having to break your concentration by reading each step of the exercise from the page.

To create an instruction tape, read the exercise number and name, then the instructions. Then play back the tape with the photos in front of you, performing the steps as they're described. You can either allow appropriate silence on the tape for performing the exercise, or you can keep the recorder nearby and hit the pause button while you hold or repeat the movement the required number of times. (Since this is a learning tool only, it's not essential that you allow time for the exact duration listed in the routine.)

Now it's time to get ready to tone, strengthen, and explore your body's fluid potential!

CHAPTER 8

Core and Spine

THE ABS and the spinal muscles that form the body's core are the foundation of good posture and graceful movement. Psychologically, the core and spine muscles represent your center of being, and provide the sense of a good, stable connection to the ground. As you begin to develop more mobility in your spine, you'll begin to feel more integration between upper and lower body, and a greater sense of being firmly rooted to the Earth.

Butterfly on Back

MOVEMENT FOCUS: Stillness, belly softening.

TIME: Thirty seconds.

1. Lie on your back.

2. Place the soles of your feet together, heels a few inches from your pubic bone, with your knees bent out to the side like butterfly wings.

3. Place your palms on your belly and take several long breaths into your palms.

BENEFITS: Frees hips, stretches adductor muscles, and improves circulation through hips.

BEGINNING MODIFICATION: Place a pillow under each knee for support.

ADVANCED MODIFICATION: While in Butterfly, add one minute of Breath of Fire. *(Breath of Fire: Inhale and exhale rapidly through your nose, with an emphasis on a strong exhale as you draw your navel in toward your spine.)*

MENTAL FOCUS: The way you begin your practice sets the tone for the rest of the journey. An opening posture such as this allows you to start your practice quietly and provides a chance to let go of your usual daily concerns, to draw your energy and awareness inward, and to become centered. This, in turn, allows you to move deeper into your own body's intelligence and benefit more greatly from your practice.

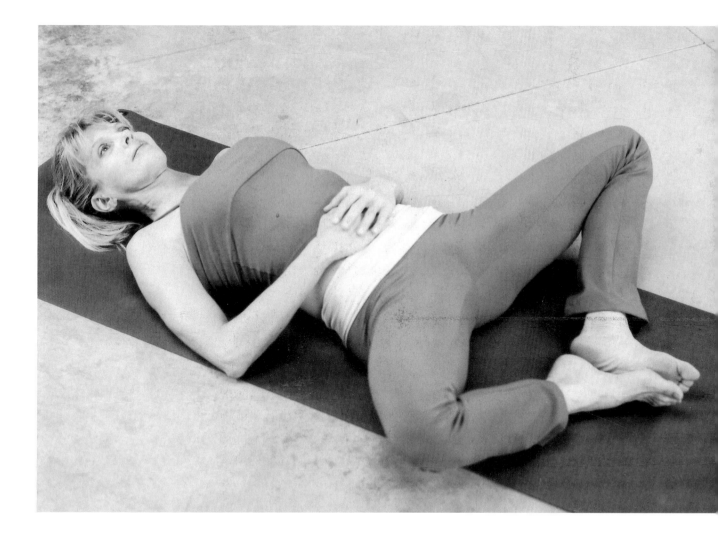

Bridge with Pelvic Tilts

Semicircular tilt in pelvis. Concentrate on contracting abdominals with exhale.

Twenty.

1. Lie on your back.

2. Bend your knees and plant your feet hip distance apart, a few inches below your sitbones.

3. Lift your hips up.

4. *Exhale* as you contract your lower abdominals, tilting your pubic bone toward your navel (Cat Tilt).

5. Keeping your hips lifted, *inhale* and release the contraction, drawing your pubic bone toward your tailbone (Dog Tilt).

6. Repeat twenty times.

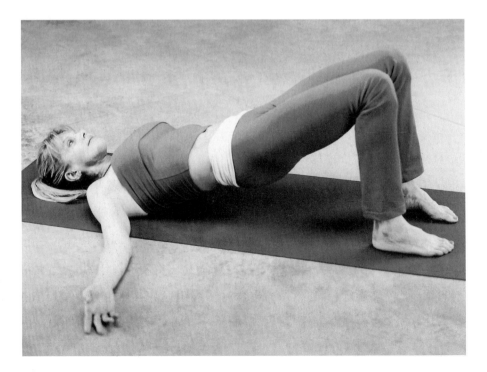

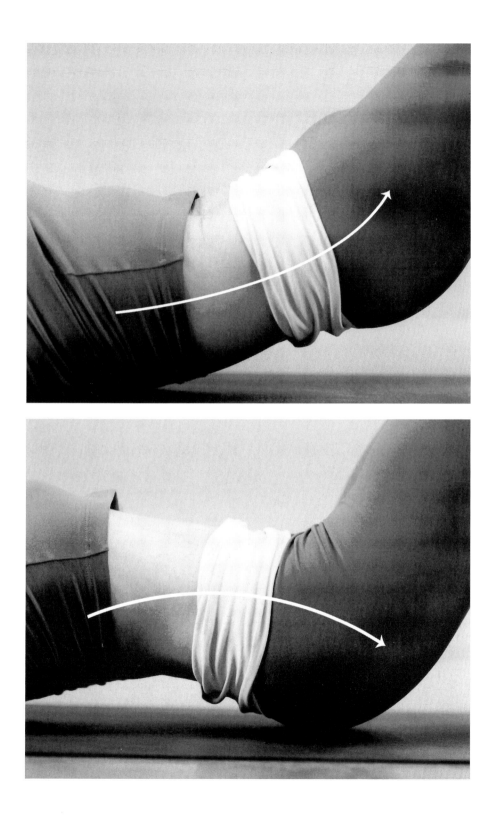

Bridge with Pelvic Circles

Circles in pelvis.

Ten in each direction.

1. Begin in the Bridge position, as on page 104.

2. Using your lower abdominals, trace a complete circle with your pubic bone.

3. Focus on initiating the movement from your core.

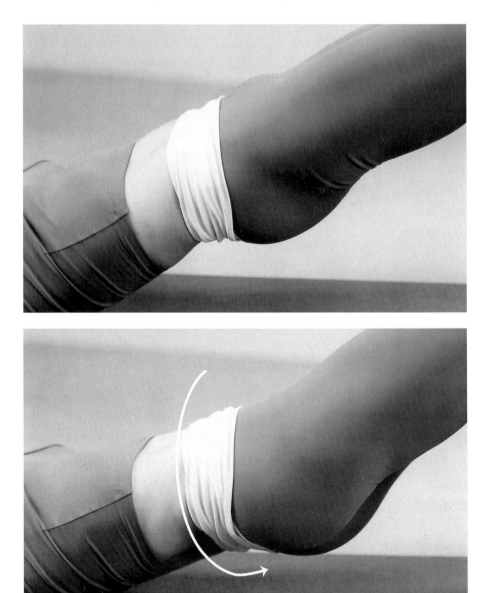

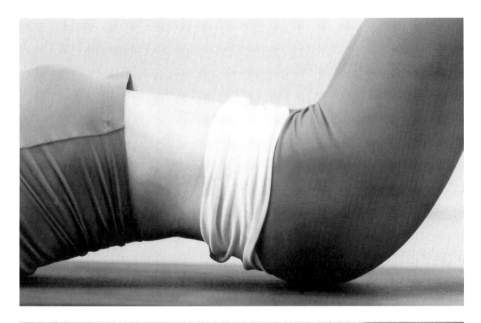

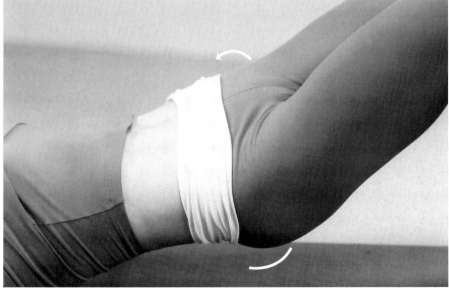

Pelvic/ Spinal Rocking

MOVEMENT FOCUS: Pelvic tilting, spinal flexion.

REPS: Twenty breaths: *Inhale* chest forward, *exhale* round back.

1. Sit in a comfortable cross-legged position.

2. Hold your ankles with both hands.

3. *Inhale,* arch your back, and lift your chest.

4. *Exhale,* bend your spine forward, rounding your back, drawing your navel toward your spine, and letting your weight shift backward slightly.

5. Keep the head movement controlled so your head does not flip-flop loosely back and forth.

MENTAL FOCUS: Keep breathing as you notice any deep-seated emotional discomfort that may arise.

BENEFITS: Draws energy up your spine and tones reproductive organs.

BEGINNING MODIFICATION: Place your fingertips a little wider than shoulder distance apart behind your back and lift your sternum. If you're uncomfortable sitting on the floor, you can do the exercise in a chair.

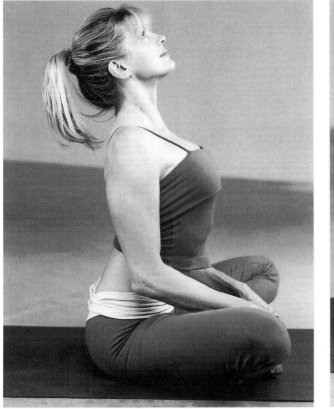

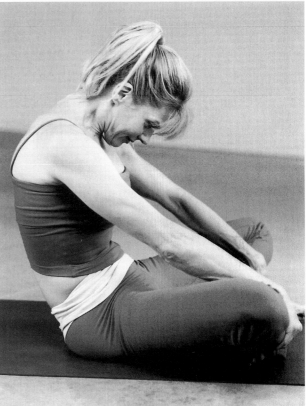

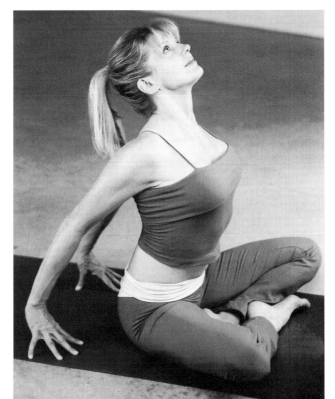

Core and Spine

Pelvic/ Spinal Rotations

MOVEMENT FOCUS: Circular movement in pelvis and spine.

REPS: Twenty breaths: *Inhale* chest forward, *exhale* round back.

1. Sit in a comfortable cross-legged position, hands resting on your knees, or place fingertips a little wider than shoulder distance apart behind you.

2. Close your eyes and focus inward.

3. Start rotating your pelvis and spine clockwise, moving your entire upper body in a circle.

4. *Inhale* as you reach your chest forward, chin extending, stretching through the throat. *Exhale* as you round your spine, chin drawing into your chest. *Breathe slowly and deeply.*

MENTAL FOCUS: Focus on serpentine movement in your core.

BENEFITS: Stimulates cerebrospinal fluid and dramatically opens up the range of motion in your spine. Very calming and sensual. Helps draw awareness inward to the sensation of the core.

BEGINNING MODIFICATION: Sit in a chair.

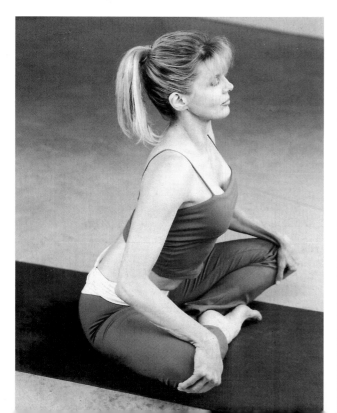
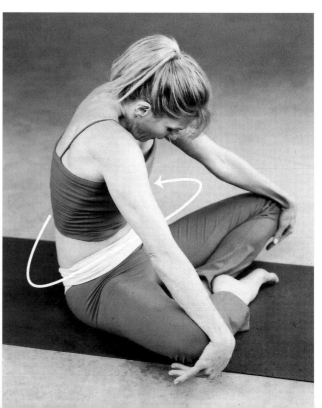

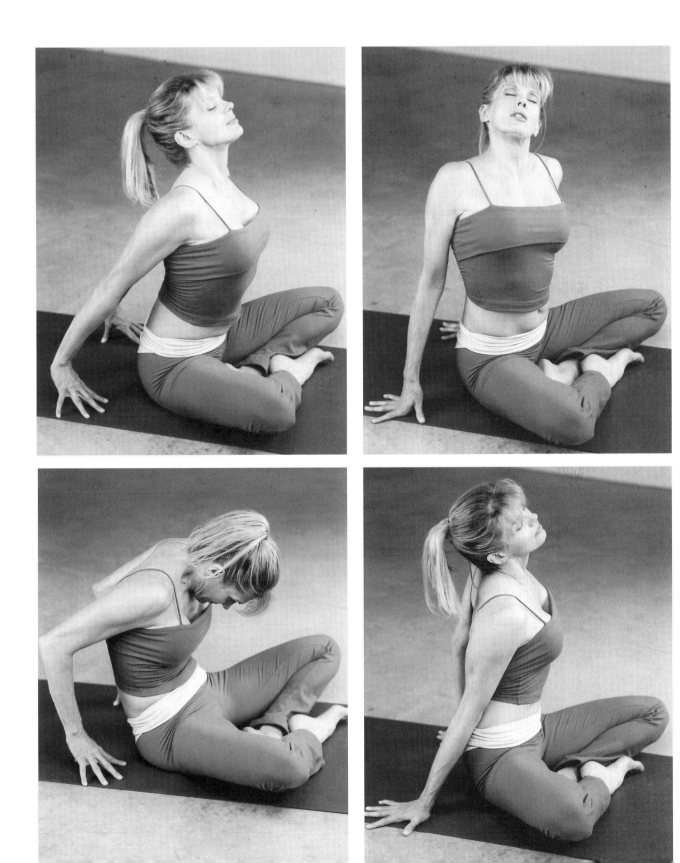

Spinal Twist

MOVEMENT FOCUS: Stillness.

TIME: Thirty seconds on each side.

1. From a seated position with legs straight in front of you, bend your right knee until the right foot is flat on the floor.

2. Lift upward along the sides of your ribs to elongate the torso. As you do so, twist to the right, bend your left elbow, and hook it over the outer right knee.

3. Place your right hand behind you for support.

4. With each breath, relax and deepen the stretch.

5. Hold for thirty seconds.

6. Switch sides and repeat.

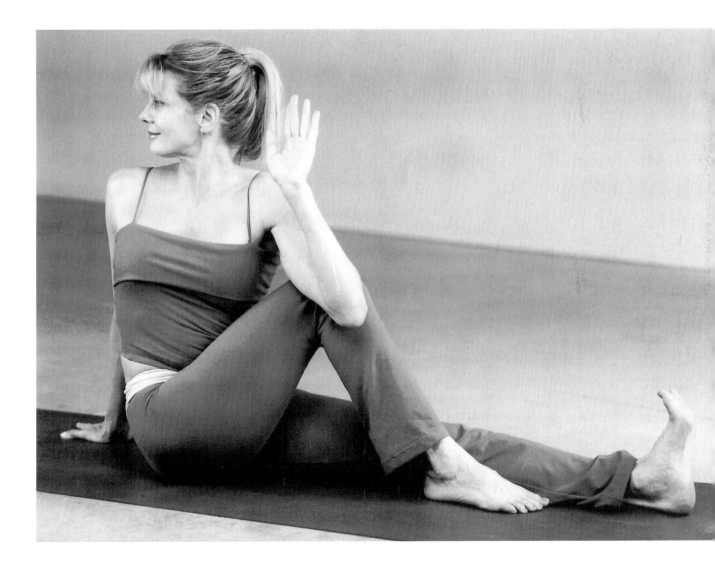

Floor Chair

Navel moves into spine; lower back into floor.

One minute.

1. Lie on your back, knees raised and bent at ninety degrees, as though you were sitting in a chair. Your knees should be hip distance apart, shins parallel to the floor.

2. Pull your navel to your spine and press your lower back into the floor.

3. Keep your breath smooth and steady.

4. Relax your shoulders, neck, and facial muscles.

BENEFITS: Strengthens and tones your core.

ADVANCED MODIFICATION: Press your palms against the tops of your thighs while resisting the pressure with your thigh muscles.

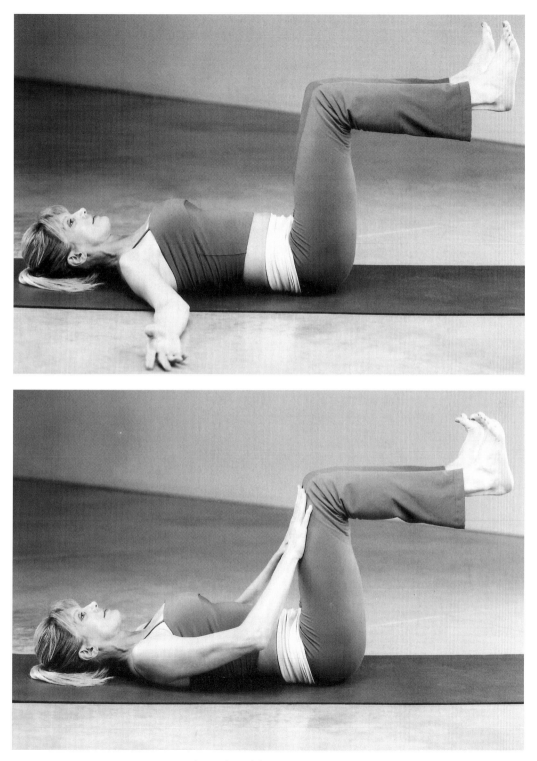

Advanced Modification

115

Floor Chair with Alternating Elbow to Knee

MOVEMENT FOCUS: Navel moves into spine; lower back into floor.

REPS: Ten on each side.

1. Begin in the same position as in Floor Chair (page 114).

2. Place your hands behind your head.

3. *Exhale* as you draw your left elbow toward your right knee.

4. Keep your right knee where it is just above your right hip. Resist the temptation to draw the knee in. Press your lower back into the floor.

5. Try to lift both shoulder blades off the floor as you contract your lower abdominals.

6. *Inhale,* bringing your shoulder blades back down to the floor.

7. *Exhale* while lifting to the other side.

BENEFITS: Strengthens and tones core.

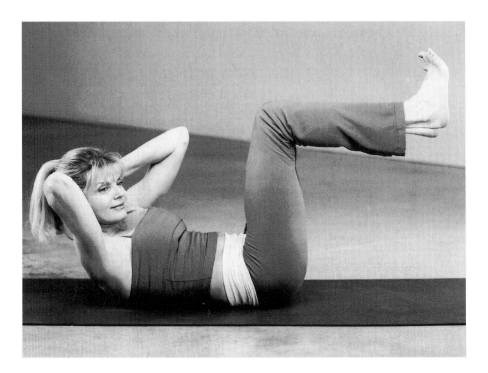

MOVEMENT FOCUS: Navel moves into spine; lower back into floor.

REPS: Ten on each side.

1. Begin as in Floor Chair with Alternating Elbow to Knee (page 116).

2. Keep your left arm straight as you *exhale* and draw it to your outer right knee.

3. Keep your knee stacked above your hip, and your lower back pressing into the floor.

4. *Inhale.* Bring your shoulder blades back down to the floor.

5. *Exhale* to the other side—left arm straight to your outer right knee.

BENEFITS: Strengthens and tones core.

Floor Chair with Alternating Straight Arm to Knee

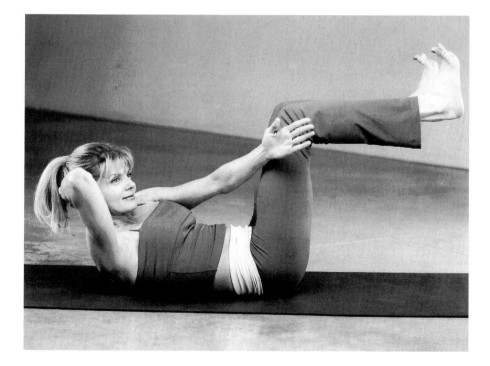

Reclining Knees to Chest

TIME: Thirty seconds.

1. Lie on your back and bring both knees into your chest.

2. *Inhale.* Elongate your entire spine, from your tailbone through the crown of your head.

3. *Exhale,* drawing your knees deeper into your chest, and pressing your lower back into the floor.

4. Feel the release in your lumbar spine and a gentle firming in your lower abdominal muscles.

5. *Inhale.* Elongate your spine.

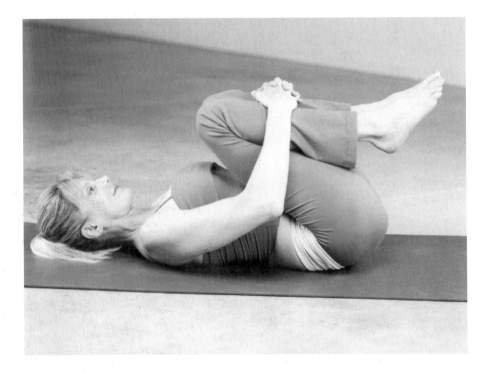

MOVEMENT FOCUS: Power spirals in spine; navel moves into spine.

TIME: Two minutes.

1. Lie on your back.

2. Draw your knees to your chest and interlace your hands behind your head.

3. *Exhale,* drawing your left elbow and right knee together while straightening your left leg to forty-five degrees.

4. Round your spine, strongly contracting your lower abdominals as you draw your pubic bone toward your navel.

5. *Inhale,* coming back to center. Lower your shoulders and bring both knees into your chest.

6. *Exhale* as you repeat on the other side.

7. Alternate sides, focusing on fluid, smooth transitions between sides.

BENEFITS: Strengthens and tones core with fluid transitions.

Core Bicycle with Alternating Elbow to Knee

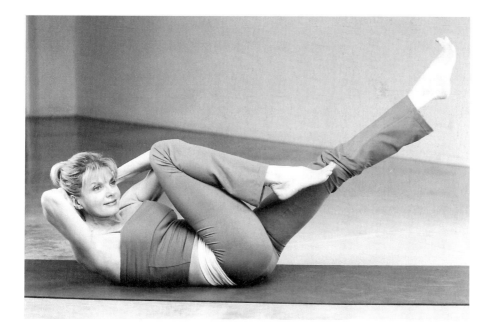

Core Bicycle with Alternating Straight Arm to Knee

Power spirals in spine; navel moves into spine.

TIME: One minute, then pulse for ten breaths at the top.

1. Begin the Core Bicycle as on page 119.

2. As you cycle, extend the opposite arm to the outside of the bent knee.

3. Focus on lifting both shoulder blades off the floor as you contract your lower abdominals, pressing your lower back into the floor.

4. Repeat for one minute and then pulse for ten breaths at the top, keeping your arm extended to the outside of your knee.

BENEFITS: Strengthens and tones core with fluid transitions.

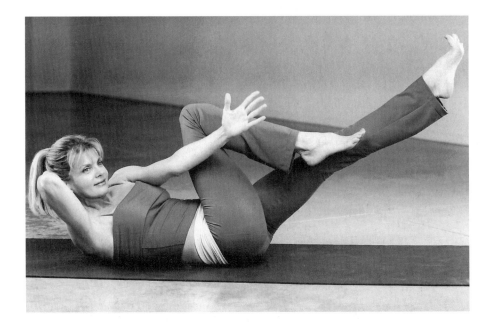

MOVEMENT FOCUS: Power spirals; navel moves into spine.

REPS: Ten on each side.

1. Begin the Core Bicycle as on page 119.

2. Keep your lower back pressed into the floor and straighten both legs to the sky.

3. *Exhale,* lowering your left leg until it is two inches off the floor. Draw your straight left arm to the outside of the straight right leg, lifting your upper torso off the floor. Keep your right leg up to the sky.

4. *Inhale,* lowering your upper torso to the floor and straightening *both* legs to the sky again.

5. Repeat ten times, alternating sides.

BENEFITS: Strengthens and tones core with fluid transitions.

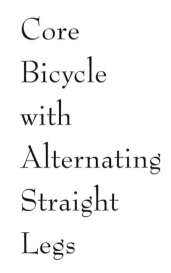

Core
Bicycle
with
Alternating
Straight
Legs

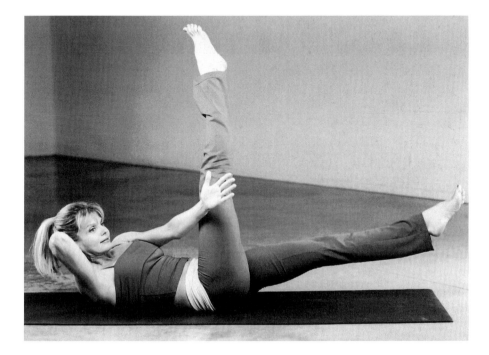

Happy Baby Pose

MOVEMENT FOCUS: Stillness; knees and lower back move into the Earth.

TIME: Thirty seconds.

1. As in Reclining Knees to Chest (page 118), lie on your back and bring both knees into your chest.

2. Move your knees apart in line with your shoulders.

3. Place your hands to the outsides of your feet.

4. *Inhale.* Elongate your entire spine, from your tailbone through the crown of your head.

5. *Exhale,* draw your knees along the sides of your torso, and press your lower back into the floor.

6. Keep your lower back and sacrum moving into the floor.

BENEFITS: Releases groins and lower back.

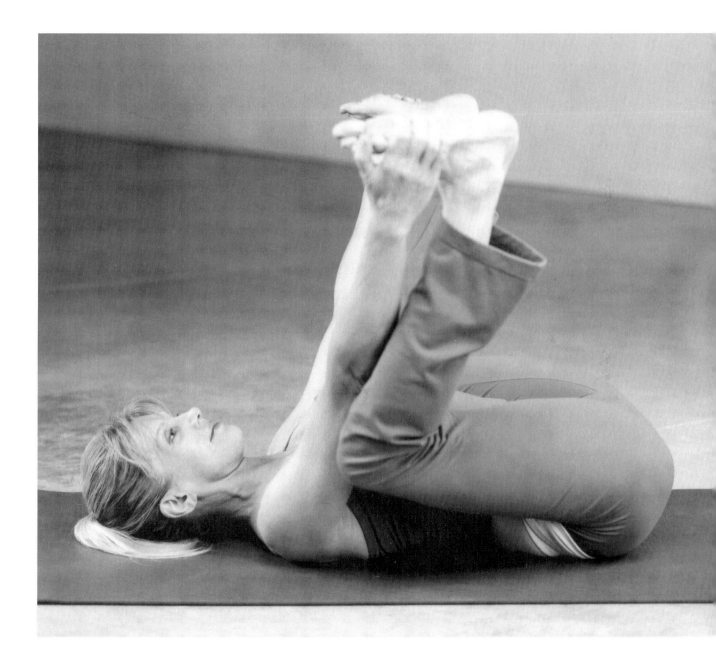

Power Core A

MOVEMENT FOCUS: Power spirals in spine; navel moves into spine.

TIME: Two minutes.

1. Lie down on your back.

2. Lift your shoulder blades and legs two inches up from the floor, keeping your chin tucked in.

3. Curl your pubic bone toward your navel and reach your arms toward your feet, parallel to the floor.

4. Start Breath of Fire as you move your arms up and down three inches, synchronized with your breath. *(Breath of Fire: Inhale and exhale rapidly through your nose, with an emphasis on a strong exhale as you draw your navel in toward your spine.)*

5. Keep your shoulder blades off the floor while pressing your navel to your lower back, and your lower back into the floor.

BENEFITS: Total core empowerment.

BEGINNING MODIFICATION: Bend your knees and place both feet on the floor, hip distance apart, eight inches away from your sitbones.

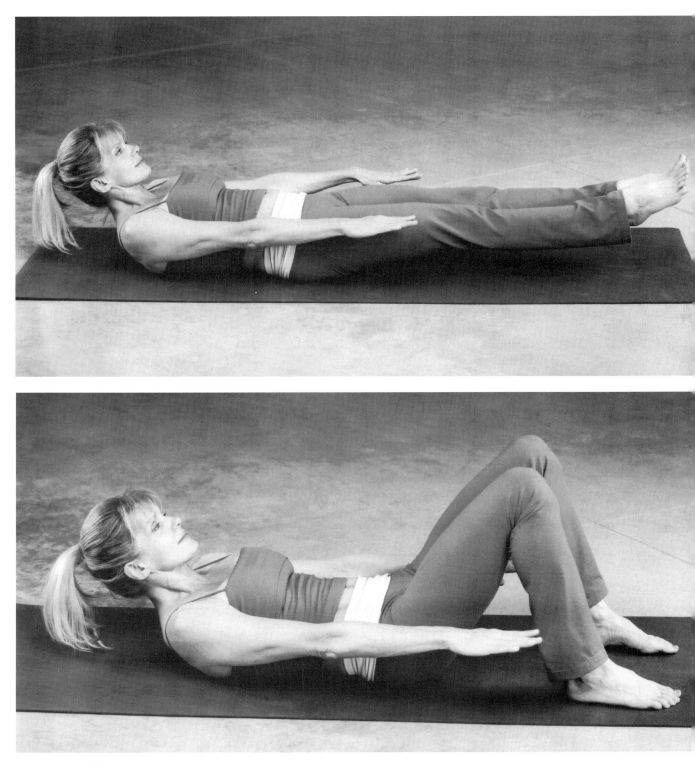

Beginning Modification

Power Core B

Power spirals in spine; navel moves into spine.

REPS: Ten lifts plus ten pulses at the top.

1. Lie on your back.

2. Lift your shoulder blades up from the floor, keeping your chin tucked in.

3. Curl your pubic bone toward your navel.

4. Keeping your navel pressing toward your spine and into the floor, straighten your legs out to the sides in a straddle.

5. Touch your palms together as you straighten your arms; *exhale,* reaching your arms through your inner thighs.

6. *Inhale,* lowering back down.

COMMENTS: The focus here is on strengthening your lower abdominals while keeping your face and jaw relaxed.

BENEFITS: Total core empowerment.

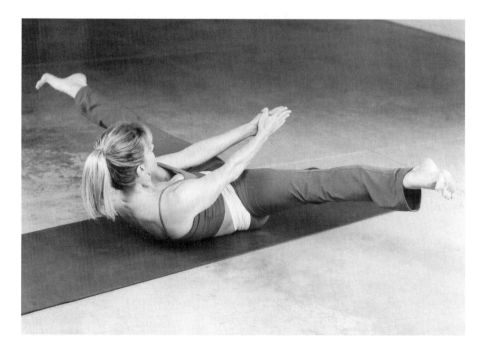

MOVEMENT FOCUS: Stillness; lower back moves into the Earth.

TIME: One minute.

1. As in Reclining Knees to Chest (page 118), lie on your back and bring both knees into your chest.

2. Grasp your knees on the outside.

3. Let the weight of your arms draw your knees out to the sides.

4. *Inhale* and *exhale* slowly, focusing on the release of your inner thighs and groins.

5. Keep your lower back and sacrum pressed into the floor.

BENEFITS: Releases groins and lower back.

Reclining Frog

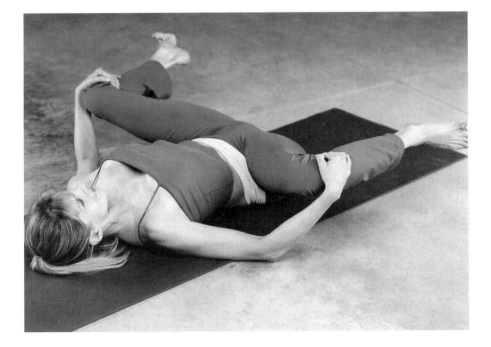

Low Lunge with Hands on Floor

Stillness; tailbone moving toward the Earth.

REPS: Ten breaths on each side.

1. Begin on your hands and knees.

2. Draw your right foot forward between your hands.

3. Keep your hands on the floor.

4. Release your tailbone down toward the floor.

5. Reach your right knee forward as you pull your left foot back.

6. Allow your neck to elongate.

7. *Inhale* and *exhale* slowly, focusing on the release of your groins and stretch of your thigh.

8. Take ten breaths and switch sides.

BENEFITS: Releases and elongates lower abdominal, hip, inner groin, and quadriceps muscles.

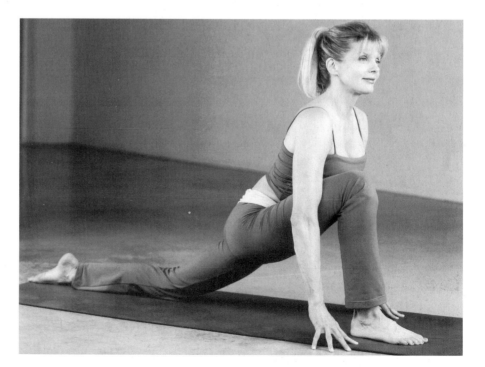

MOVEMENT FOCUS: Stillness; internal elongation of spine.

TIME: Ten breaths on each side.

1. Perform the Lunge as on page 128.

2. Take your arms up.

3. Lift your lower belly and entire rib cage up and off your pelvis.

4. Extend your front and back body evenly.

5. Relax your shoulders down away from your ears as you powerfully elongate and lift your spine to the sky.

6. Take ten breaths, then release and repeat on the other side.

BENEFITS: Releases, strengthens, and elongates your entire spine and core as well as your groin (psoas) and thighs. Tones core and back muscles.

Low Lunge with Arms Up

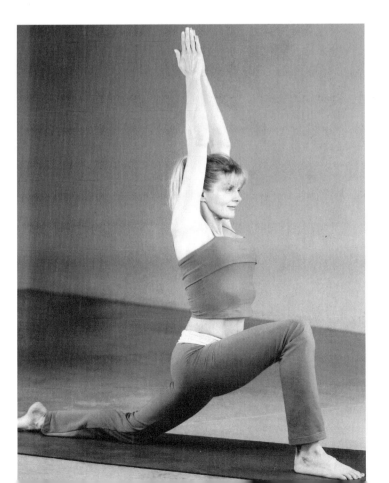

Crescent Moon with Arms Up

MOVEMENT FOCUS: Stillness; internal elongation of spine.

TIME: Ten breaths on each side.

1. Begin in the Lunge position on page 128.

2. Curl your back toes under and lift your back knee off the floor.

3. Stretch your arms up overhead and lift your upper torso toward the sky.

4. Reach up farther by hooking your thumbs together and spreading your fingers.

5. Soften the muscles around your neck and face.

6. Move your right knee forward as you pull your left heel back.

7. Lift your rib cage off your pelvis.

8. Take ten breaths, then relax and repeat on the other side.

BENEFITS: Releases, strengthens, and elongates your entire spine and core muscles, groin (psoas), and thigh muscles.

BEGINNING MODIFICATION: Keep your hands on your front thigh, close to your knee, for extra support.

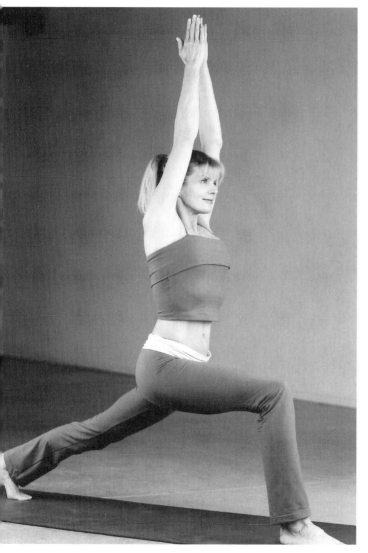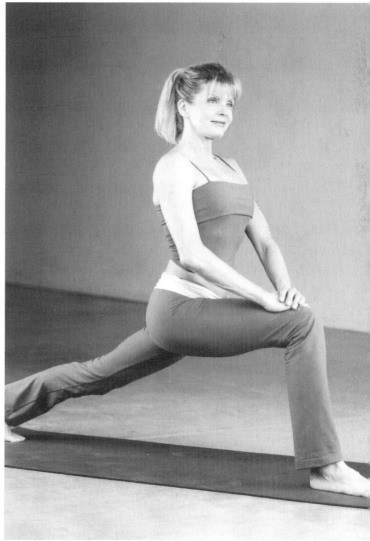

Beginning Modification

Child's Pose

MOVEMENT FOCUS: Melting shoulders around knees; stillness.

TIME: Thirty seconds.

1. Begin on your hands and knees, with your knees and shins together.

2. Keeping your hands on the floor, sit back, drawing your sitbones toward your heels.

3. Lay your chest onto your thighs and place your forehead on the floor.

4. Place your hands, palms up, by your feet.

5. Wrap your shoulders around your knees and allow them to release, melting like wax around your knees.

BENEFITS: Child's Pose relaxes, releases, and grounds all at once. It is a rejuvenating posture that helps us draw our awareness inward in a calm, effortless way.

NOTE: If you have any knee pain, place a bed pillow behind your knees to support them.

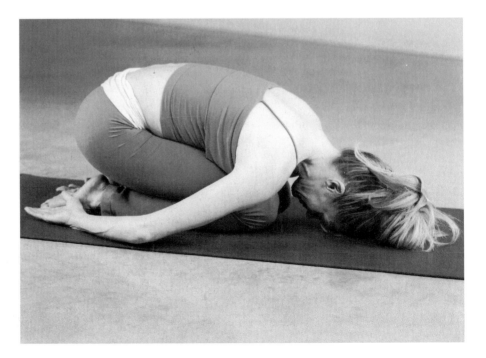

MOVEMENT FOCUS: Stillness; internal elongation of spine.

REPS: Ten; *inhale* up, *exhale* down.

1. Lie facedown with your arms alongside your body, palms and forehead down.

2. Pull your navel toward your spine, pressing your pubic bone firmly into the floor to give length to your lower spine.

3. Stretch each foot back as far as you can, creating a line of energy through each leg.

4. Pull your shoulders up away from the floor and down away from your ears.

5. *Inhale* and lift your upper body away from the floor.

6. *Exhale* as you lower your upper body back onto the floor.

7. Move in a smooth, fluid way as you rise and melt back into the floor.

8. Keep your hands and feet on the floor.

BENEFITS: Strengthens back and core.

Locust with Hands Behind Back

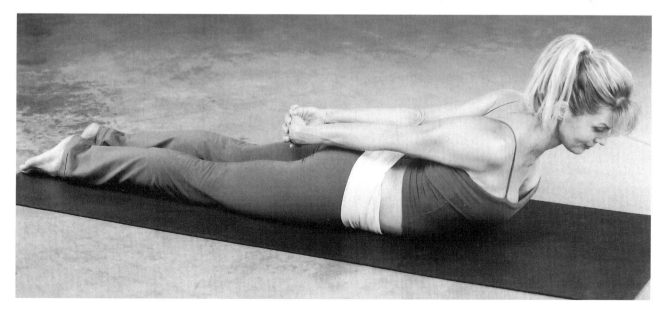

Locust Dance with Arm Movement

MOVEMENT FOCUS: Semicircle; wave in spine extending through body.

REPS: Ten; *inhale* up, *exhale* down.

1. Lie facedown with your arms stretched above your head.

2. Focus on moving smoothly with your breath.

3. On the *inhalation:*

   ➤ Lift your chest.

   ➤ Lift your arms a couple of inches and stretch them forward in front of you.

   ➤ Stretch and lift your legs up off the floor.

4. On the *exhalation,* reverse the movement:

   ➤ Lower your chest and arms to the floor.

   ➤ Lower your legs.

5. Synchronize these movements with your breath in a smooth, fluid way.

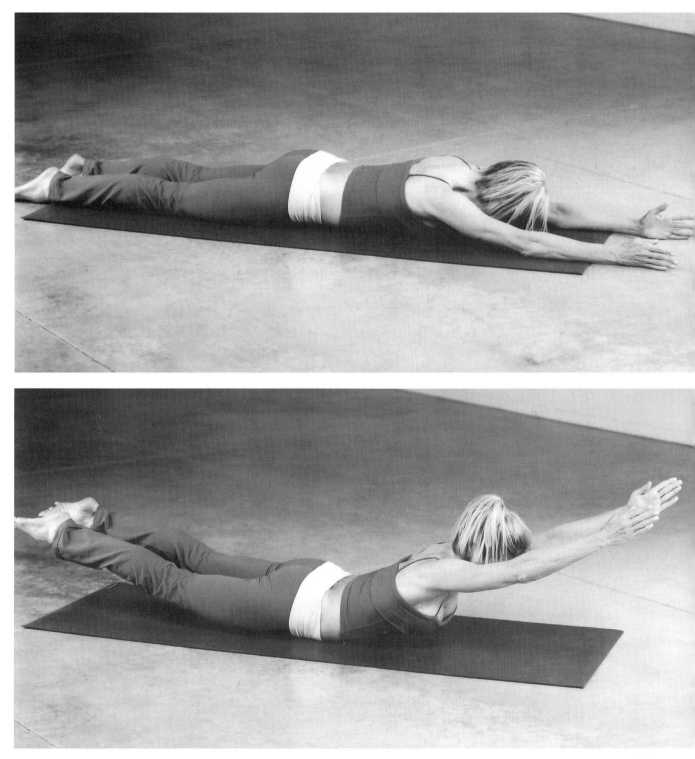

Cobra

Stillness; internal elongation of spine.

TIME: Ten breaths.

1. As in Locust pose (page 133), lie on your belly, forehead on the floor. Place your palms alongside your breasts, fingertips in line with your shoulders.

2. Lift your abdominal muscles inward toward your spine and press your pubic bone into the floor. Press into the tops of your feet and stretch back through each foot.

3. Roll your shoulders down away from your ears, drawing the bottom tips of the shoulder blades toward each other. Feel your chest open as you do this.

4. Inhale as you raise your upper torso away from the floor, keeping your elbows in toward your rib cage.

5. Make sure to keep your legs on the floor, your sitbones reaching toward your heels.

6. Take ten breaths.

BENEFITS: Opens chest and upper spine. Increases strength and flexibility of spine and back. Improves lung capacity, digestion, elimination.

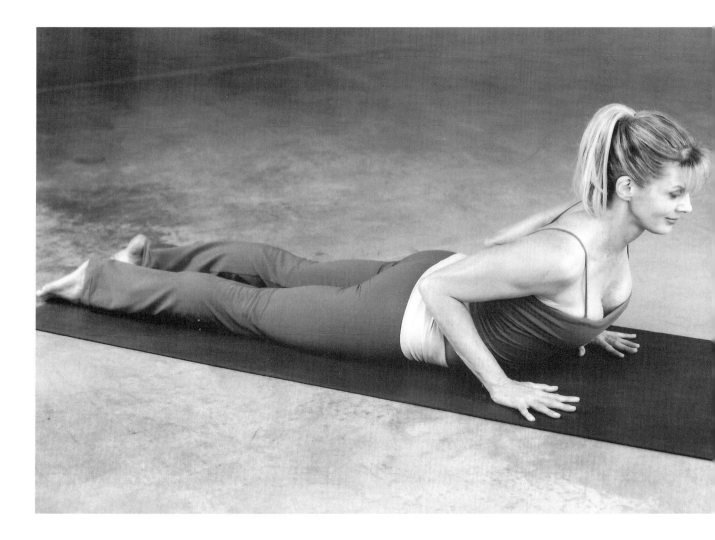

Cobra Dance

MOVEMENT FOCUS: Wave movement in spine.

REPS: Ten.

1. Begin as in Cobra (page 136) with forehead on the floor.

2. *Inhale* as you lift your upper torso.

3. *Exhale,* lowering your upper torso.

4. With each inhale, lift your torso higher and higher, curving up as far as you comfortably can without any strain in your lower back and without using your hands to lift your torso.

5. Let your movement come from your center in accord with your breath.

6. Allow a smooth, wavelike movement in your spine as you lift and lower it.

7. Notice how the center of the curve moves down your back as you move deeper into the pose—from your upper back, to the middle back, to your lumbar spine.

8. Eventually, you can straighten your arms, keeping your shoulders down away from your ears.

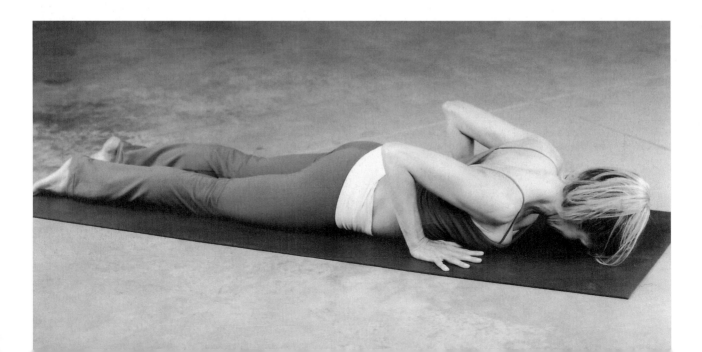

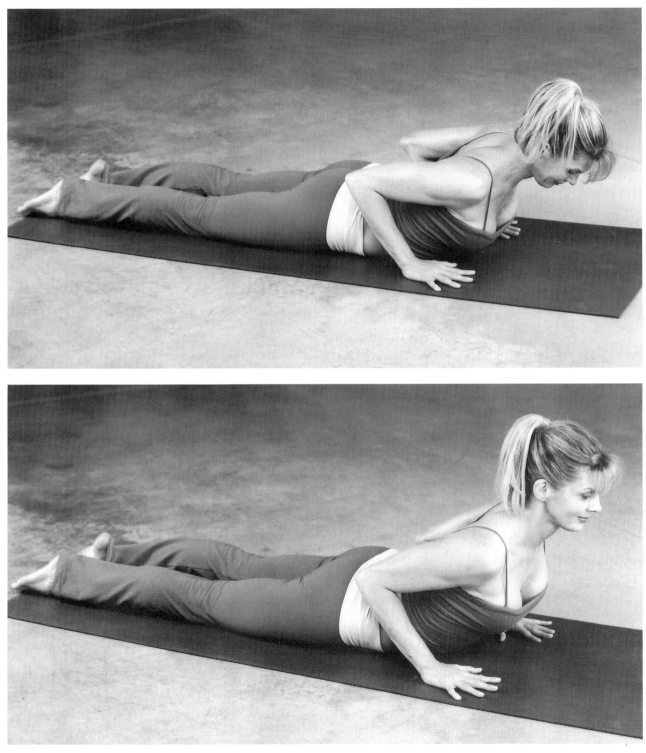

Boat Pose

Stillness; internal elongation of spine.

TIME: Forty-five seconds.

1. Lie down on your belly.

2. Bend your knees and clasp your ankles from the outside with each hand.

3. Lift your lower belly into your spine.

4. Draw your tailbone toward your pubic bone and lift your inner thighs up toward the ceiling.

5. *Inhale,* lifting your upper body away from the floor.

6. *Exhale,* lifting your feet higher and spreading your toes. Keep your face relaxed.

7. Keep elongating the back of your neck as well as your lower back.

BENEFITS: Builds tremendous strength and elasticity in the spine. Elongates chest, shoulders, abdominals. Tones abdominal organs and stimulates kidneys and adrenals.

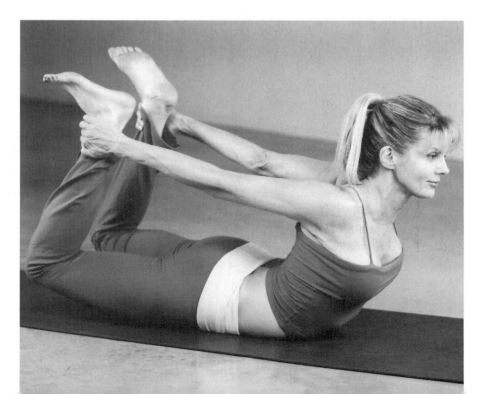

MOVEMENT FOCUS: Stillness.

TIME: Ten breaths on each side.

1. Lie down on your left side, resting on a straight arm, with your wrist under your shoulder.

2. Stack (align) your hips, knees, and ankles, and flex your feet.

3. Release the left side of your rib cage toward the floor as you press out through both heels.

4. Place your other hand on the floor in front of you to help stay balanced and aligned.

5. Hold for ten breaths; switch sides and repeat.

BEGINNING MODIFICATION: Rest on your forearm.

Alligator Stretch

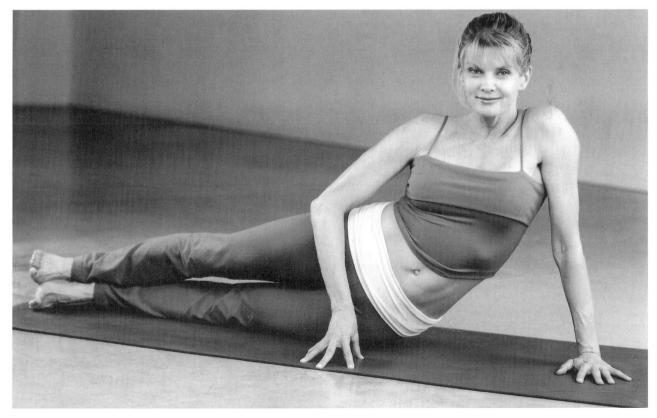

Belly to Earth Meditation

MOVEMENT FOCUS: Stillness.

TIME: One minute.

1. Lie facedown, allowing your bones and muscles to melt into the floor.

2. Cross your forearms and place your forehead on your forearms.

3. Relax your facial muscles, neck, and shoulders.

4. Enjoy the feeling of your belly and the belly of the Earth meeting.

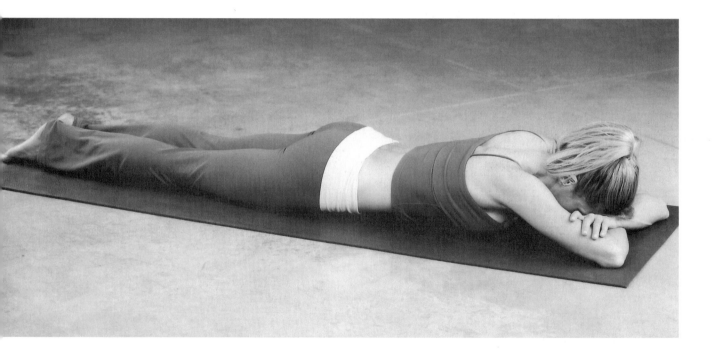

MOVEMENT FOCUS: Pelvis rocks side to side.

TIME: Thirty seconds.

1. Begin in the pose on page 142.

2. Wiggle your hips side to side.

BENEFITS: Helps release bound-up energy in the lower back and pelvis, allowing it to flow more freely.

Belly to Earth with Puppy Tail

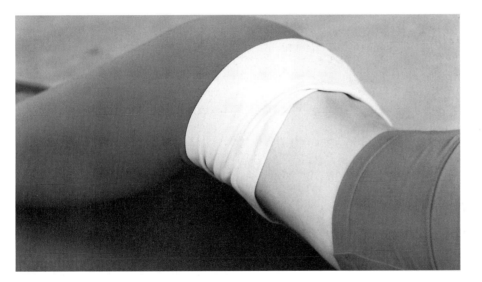

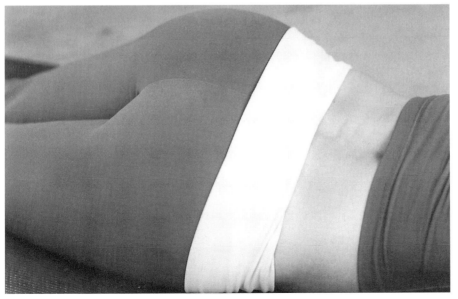

Belly to Earth Caterpillar

Pelvic tilts, rippling wave movement in spine.

One minute.

1. Begin as on page 142.

2. Add a pelvic tilt motion: *Exhale* as you strongly contract your abdominals, curling your pubic bone toward your navel (Cat Tilt); *inhale* as you slightly relax the contraction and lift your pubic bone back toward your tailbone (Dog Tilt).

3. Allow this pelvic motion to send a rippling wave up your spine, all the way to the crown of your head.

4. As one wave ends, the next begins, in a continuous, liquid movement. *Imagine a caterpillar walking along the floor.*

5. Focus on initiating the movement from the base of your spine and pelvis.

6. Don't get frustrated if your movement seems choppy at first. Be patient and keep feeling into how your breath and spine meet.

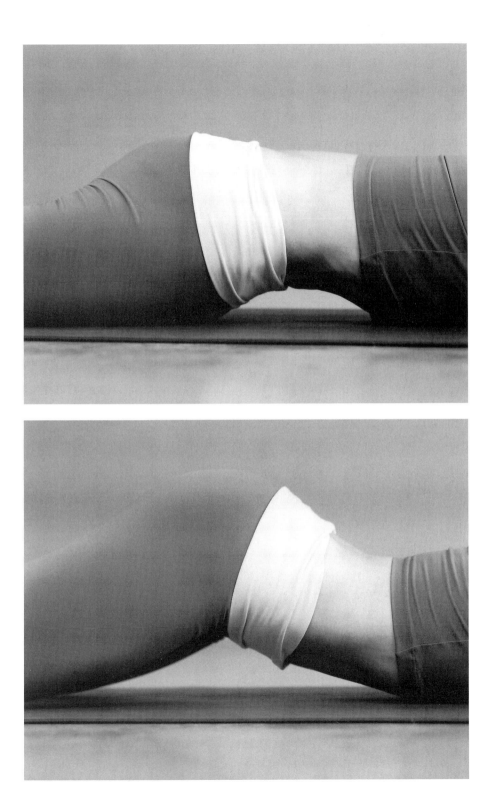

Cat's Breath

Semicircular flexion in spine.

Ten slow cycles and ten fast cycles.

1. Start on your hands and knees.

2. Place your hands directly beneath your shoulders with the middle finger forward and your knees directly beneath your hips.

3. Establish a smooth, flowing ujjayi breath in the back of your throat.

4. Create a line of energy in each arm by pressing down, elongating your arms and spine from your tailbone to the crown of your head.

5. *Exhale,* tucking your hips into Cat Tilt by drawing your belly in and rounding your back.

6. Firm your buttocks as you pull your tailbone and forehead toward each other.

7. *Inhale,* reversing the motion into a Dog Tilt: Soften your belly and lift your head, chest, and sitbones upward, rocking your pelvis down and back.

8. Keep pressing down into your arms, lifting out of your shoulders as you open your chest.

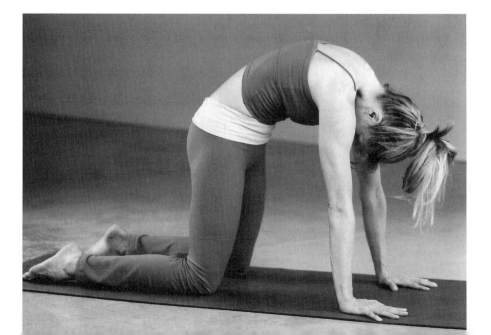

9. Create a smooth, arching curve in your lower back as you continue to draw your navel toward your spine and reach your sitbones upward.

10. Gently rock back and forth between Cat and Dog Tilt.

BENEFITS: Cat's Breath Series teaches you to initiate movement from your center and to synchronize the movement of your breath with the movement of your body, specifically your spine. These exercises will stimulate the circulation of cerebrospinal fluid, which nourishes and plumps up the supportive disks between the vertebrae to create a more flexible, healthy spine. They're great to do if you are feeling dull, sluggish, or distracted.

NOTE: If necessary, place extra padding under your knees for extra support.

MENTAL FOCUS:

> Enjoy the fluid, sensual quality of your spine, and the sensation of breath and spine meeting.

> Try closing your eyes to feel a more internal, sensual connection to your movement.

> If your movement feels choppy and stuck, slow down. *Imagine your spine as seaweed, flowing back and forth in the ocean's currents.*

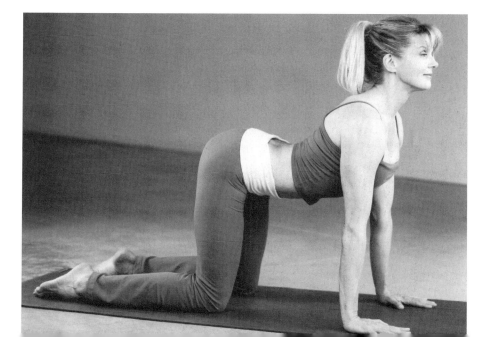

Cat's Breath Spine Dance A— On Hands and Knees

MOVEMENT FOCUS: Circles and waves in spine.

TIME: One minute in each direction.

1. Start on your hands and knees.

2. Place your hands directly beneath your shoulders with the middle finger forward and your knees directly beneath your hips.

3. Establish a smooth, flowing ujjayi breath in the back of your throat.

4. Create a line of energy in each arm by pressing down, elongating your arms and spine from your tailbone to the crown of your head.

5. Create a circular movement in your rib cage as if it were revolving around your spine.

6. Allow the flow of movement to travel up and down your spine.

7. Feel how each circle meets your hips and spine. (You may want to take your hands and knees wider to facilitate the circular movement of the spine and hips.)

8. Close your eyes and go inside, following the fluid, delicious sensation of your spine dancing.

9. Allow the movement to become spontaneous as your spine and breath meet. Try exhaling several times through your mouth and allow your spine to sway back and forth.

10. Have fun exploring how you can move from within. *Imagine seaweed in the ocean, or a snake slithering along the ground.*

11. Continue for one minute; switch directions and repeat.

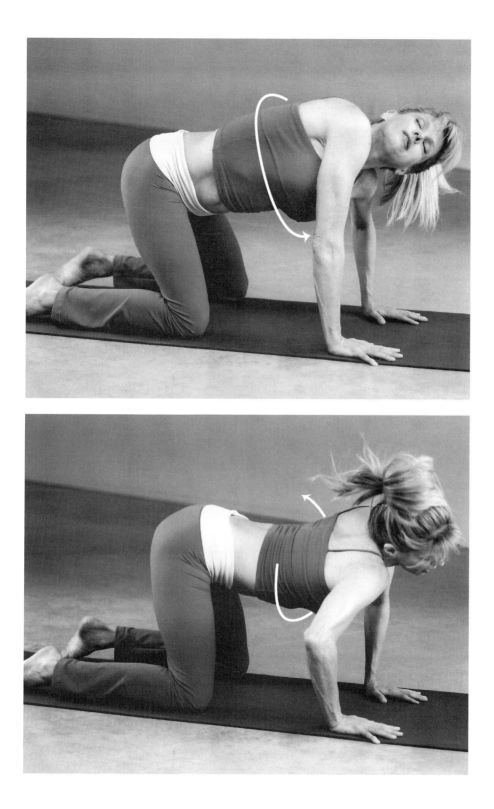

Cat's Breath Spine Dance B— Sitting

MOVEMENT FOCUS: Circles and waves in spine.

TIME: One minute in each direction.

1. Sit with your legs forward, knees bent, and feet placed two to three feet apart.

2. Place your palms down behind you to help support your spine.

3. Perform the same circular rotation of your rib cage as in Spine Dance A (page 148).

4. Allow your hips, pelvis, spine, and breath to meet through the circular, undulating movement of your core and spine.

5. Continue for one minute; switch directions and repeat.

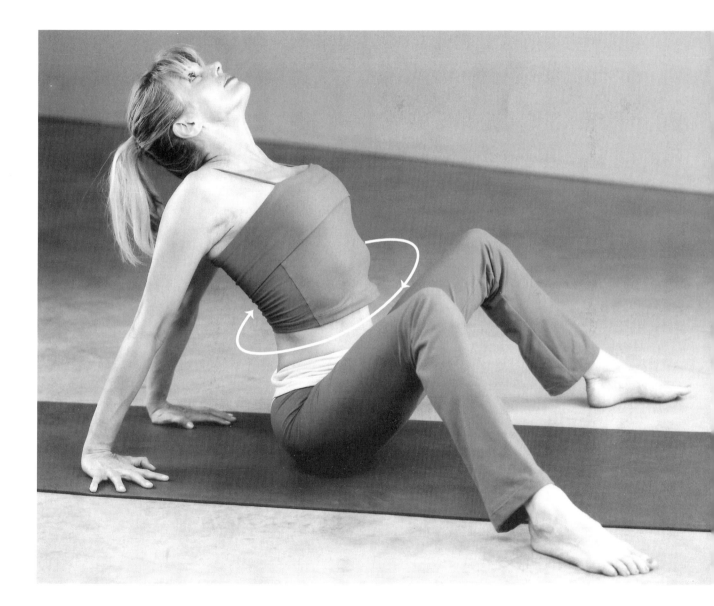

Standing Rib Cage Isolations

MOVEMENT FOCUS: Circles in spine.

REPS: Five isolated circles in each direction; ten fluid circles in each direction.

1. Stand with your feet hip distance apart.

2. Trace four points of a circle (front, right side, back, left side) with your rib cage while keeping your hips stationary.

3. Repeat five times in each direction, stopping between circles; then make ten smooth, fluid circles with your rib cage in each direction.

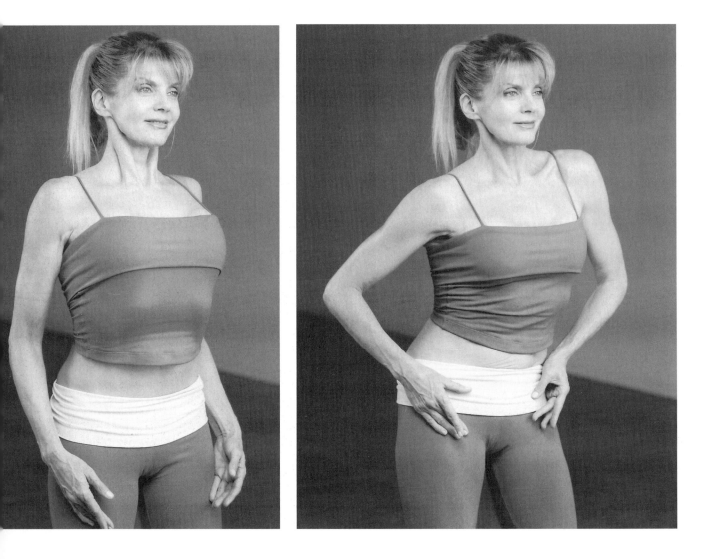

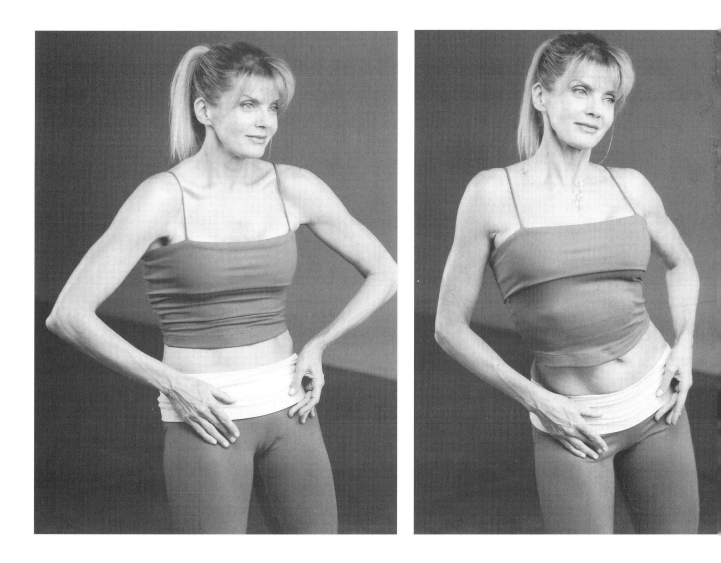

Standing Cat's Breath

MOVEMENT FOCUS: Semicircular flexion in spine.

TIME: One minute.

1. Stand with your hands placed on your midthighs.

2. As on page 146, create Cat's Breath motion in spine.

3. *Inhale* as you tilt your tailbone up and lift your head and chest.

4. *Exhale* as you reverse motion, drawing your tailbone and forehead toward each other.

5. Close your eyes and go inside, following the fluid, delicious sensation of your spine arching and rounding.

6. Allow the movement to become spontaneous as your spine and breath meet.

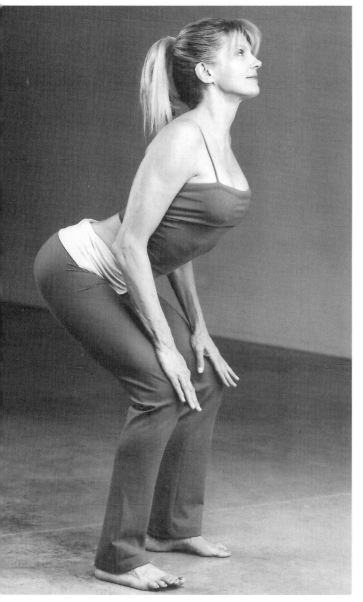
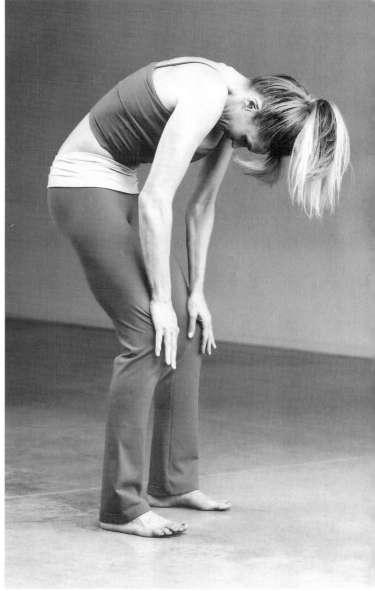

Standing Spine Dance A

MOVEMENT FOCUS: Circles and waves in spine.

TIME: One minute in each direction.

1. Stand with your hands placed on your midthighs.

2. As in Cat's Breath Spine Dance B (page 150), create a circular movement in your rib cage as if it were revolving around your spine.

3. Allow the flow of movement to travel up and down your spine.

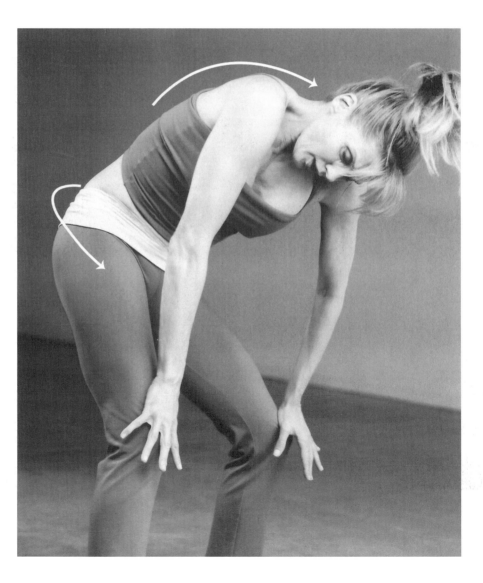

4. Feel how each circle meets your hips and spine. (You may want to take your hands and knees wider to facilitate the circular movement of your spine and hips.)

5. Close your eyes and go inside, following the fluid, delicious sensation of your spine dancing. *Imagine seaweed in the ocean, or a snake slithering along the ground.*

6. Continue for one minute; switch directions and repeat.

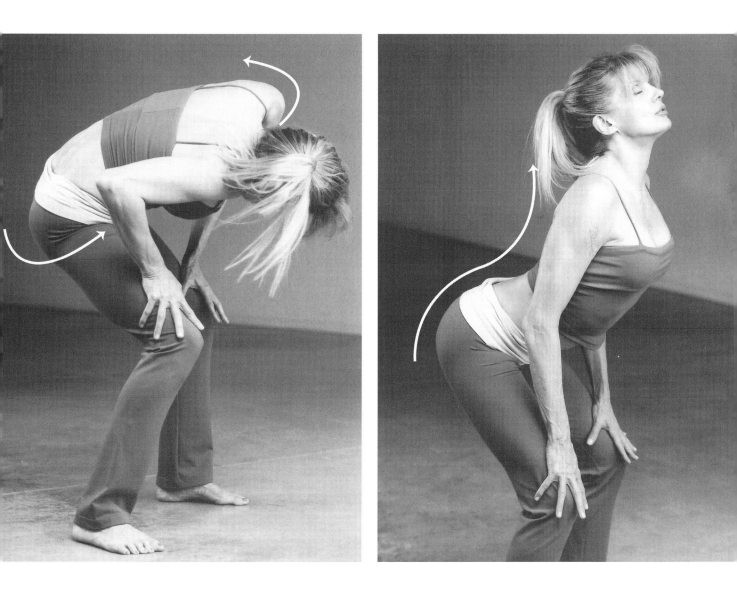

Standing Spine Dance B

MOVEMENT FOCUS: Circles and waves in spine.

TIME: Two minutes.

1. Stand facing a wall, and place your hands on the wall a little wider than shoulder distance apart.

2. As in Cat's Breath Spine Dance B (page 150), create a circular movement in your rib cage as if it were revolving around your spine.

3. Allow the flow of movement to travel up and down your spine.

4. Feel how each circle meets your hips and spine. (You may want to take your hands and knees wider to facilitate the circular movement of your spine and hips.)

5. Close your eyes and go inside, following the fluid, delicious sensation of your spine dancing.

6. Continue for two minutes; switch directions and repeat.

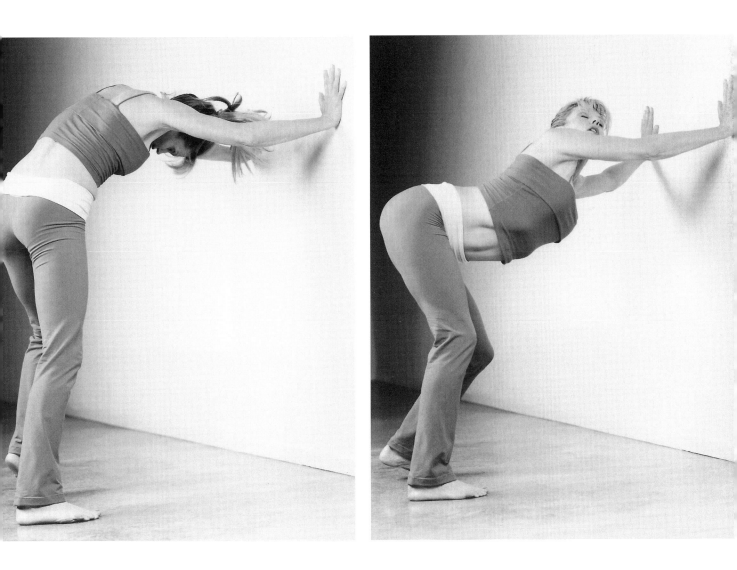

Standing Neck Release

TIME: Thirty seconds on each side.

1. Stand with your feet hip distance apart.

2. Interlace your fingers behind your back.

3. Draw both interlaced hands to your right hip, keeping your shoulders down away from your ears and drawing your elbows toward each other.

4. Lower your right ear toward your right shoulder, keeping your left shoulder down away from the ear. Feel the release of the muscles on the side of your neck as your cervical spine opens and releases.

5. Continue for thirty seconds; switch sides and repeat.

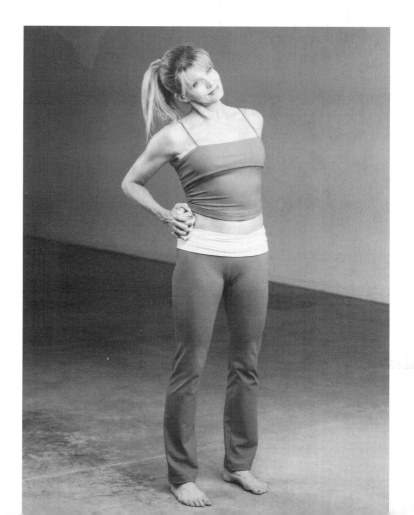

MOVEMENT FOCUS: Stillness; elongation of spine.

TIME: One minute.

1. Stand and rest your sitbones on the wall.

2. Place your feet hip distance apart, one and a half to two feet from the wall.

3. Keeping your sitbones at the wall, interlace your forearms and fold forward.

4. Focus on elongating your spine and releasing your back muscles.

Standing Forward Bend— Against Wall

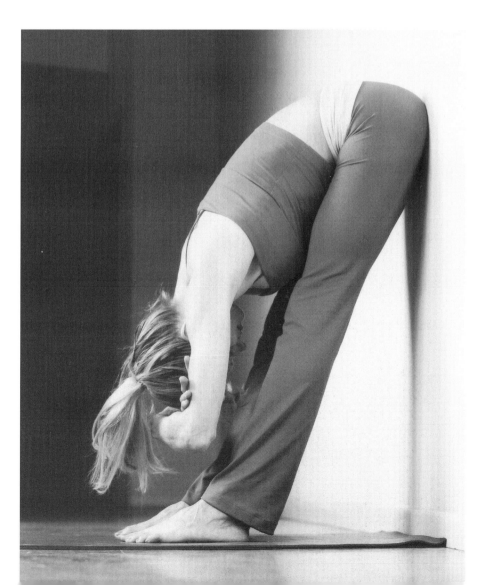

Seated Forward Bend

MOVEMENT FOCUS: Stillness; elongation of spine.

TIME: One minute.

1. Sit down on the floor, legs extended, and bring your ankles and big toes together.

2. Contract your thighs, drawing your muscles into the bone.

3. *Inhale* and stretch your spine up.

4. *Exhale* and pour yourself over your legs.

5. Focus on elongating from the base of your spine, not rounding your upper spine.

6. Feel into the release of your back body, including your hamstrings, calves, and back muscles.

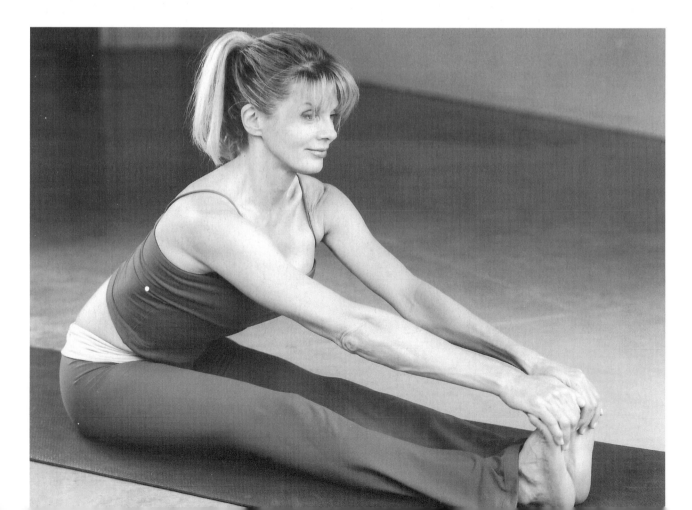

MOVEMENT FOCUS: Stillness.

TIME: Thirty seconds on each side.

1. Lie down, bend your knees, and place your feet four to six inches away from your sitbones, hip distance apart.

2. Drop your knees to the right.

3. Cross your right ankle on top of your left thigh.

4. Enjoy the sensation of release from deep inside your pelvis.

5. Hold for thirty seconds; switch sides and repeat.

BENEFITS: A great release for the psoas muscles and groin muscles.

Reclining Psoas Release

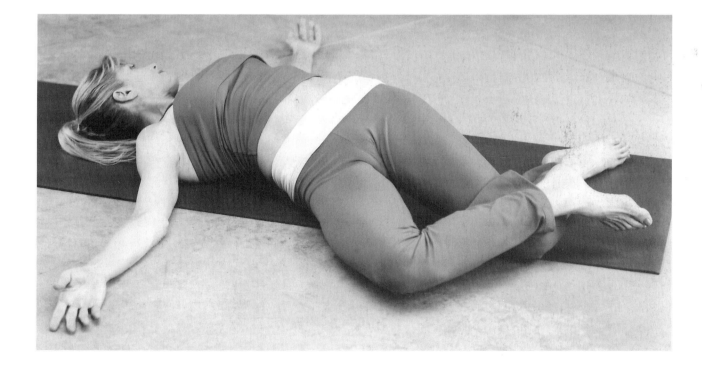

Reclining Spinal Twist

MOVEMENT FOCUS: Stillness; elongation of spine.

TIME: Thirty seconds on each side.

1. Lie down on your back and feel your back body connecting to the Earth.

2. Draw your left knee into your chest, keeping your lower back pressing into the floor. *Exhale,* drawing the bent knee across your body to the right.

3. Reach out with your left arm and look over your left shoulder.

4. *Inhale,* elongating your spine.

5. *Exhale,* deepening the twist.

6. Hold for thirty seconds; switch sides and repeat.

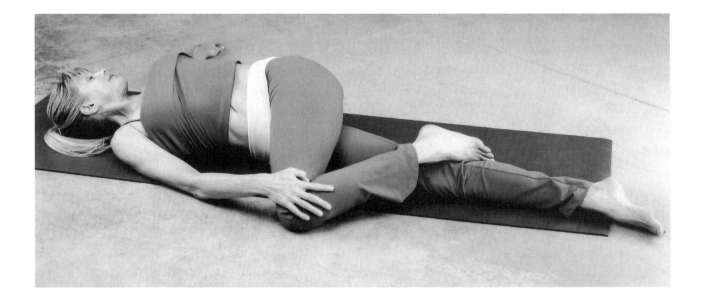

MOVEMENT FOCUS: Stillness.

TIME: Three to five minutes.

1. Lie down on your back with straight arms and legs.

2. Relax your shoulders down away from your ears. Allow the weight of your bones to surrender to the support of the Earth.

3. Allow a wave of relaxation to wash over you from the top of your head all the way to your toes.

4. Breathe softly and slowly.

5. Soften and relax your facial muscles, eyes, lips, tongue, and jaw.

Savasana Full-Body Meditation

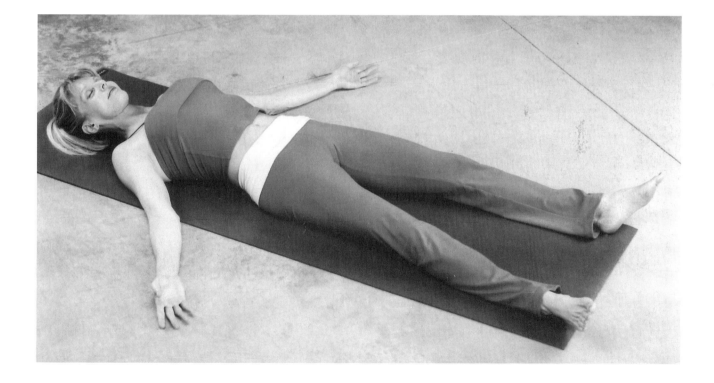

CHAPTER 9

Hips, Pelvis, and Legs

ROM A FITNESS STANDPOINT, the legs and buttocks are one of everyone's favorite areas to target for improving tone and contour. Also, being the business end of all the sitting we do during the day, the hips, buttocks, and legs are very prone to stiffness and diminished circulation.

At the same time, this area is the center of sexual power. So much of our sensuality is wrapped up in the *movement* of the hips.

The following routine is designed to integrate the muscles of this area to provide a very thorough workout, while at the same time releasing back pain, opening the hips, and stimulating and releasing sensual energy.

Reclining Knees to Chest

MOVEMENT FOCUS: Stillness, elongating spine, knees drawing to chest.

TIME: Thirty seconds.

1. Lie on your back and bring both knees into your chest.

2. Elongate your entire spine from your tailbone through the crown of your head.

3. *Exhale.* Draw your knees deeper into your chest and press your lower back into the floor, feeling the release in your lumbar spine and a gentle toning in your lower abdominal muscles.

4. *Inhale.* Elongate your spine.

MENTAL FOCUS: To center yourself, become intimately aware of your breathing. Deepen your breath with ujjayi breath *(ujjayi breath: lips closed, whisper sound in back of throat),* with an emphasis on creating a long, smooth *inhale* and *exhale.* This focus on your breath is the foundation for the rest of your practice. Focus on releasing the muscles along your back and elongating your spine as you breathe steadily and deeply.

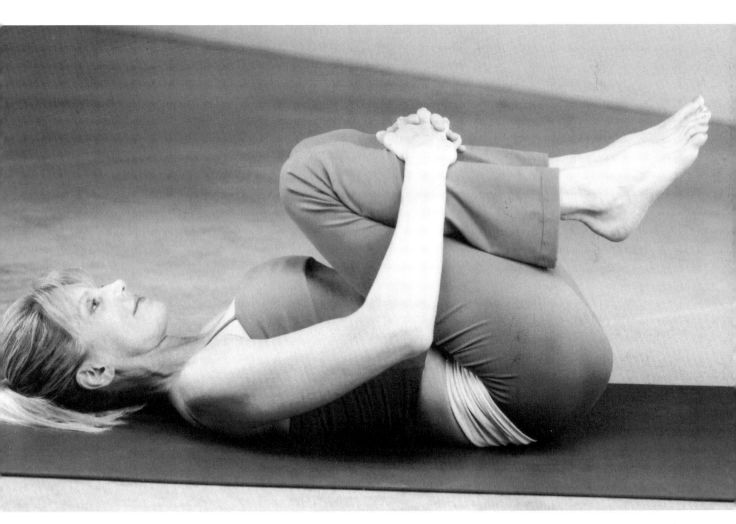

Reclining Spinal Twist

MOVEMENT FOCUS: Elongate spine on inhale; deepen twist on exhale.

TIME: One minute on each side.

1. Lie on your back with your legs straight.

2. Draw your right knee into your chest.

3. *Inhale* deeply and elongate your spine. Keep your chin in.

4. *Exhale* as you draw your right knee across the left side of your body to reach the floor.

5. Stretch your rib cage and chest away from your waist and reach out with your right arm. Turn your head to look over your right shoulder.

6. Allow the twist of the spine to deepen with each exhale.

7. Enjoy the feeling of loosening, unwinding, and letting go.

8. Hold for one minute and then switch sides.

MENTAL FOCUS: As you draw your awareness inward, feel the breath meeting your body. Soften and breathe into any areas that may feel stuck or tight. Connect to a feeling of *unfurling*.

BENEFITS: Spinal twists alleviate tremendous amounts of tension in the body. As you gently elongate and twist the spine, you will begin to feel a delicious unfurling, freedom, and mobility from your center.

NOTE: Don't do Spinal Twists if you are pregnant.

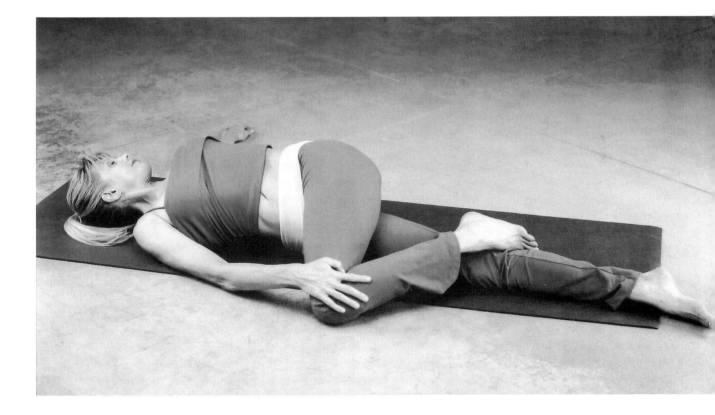

Bridge Pose Series— Hold with Kegels

Rhythmic pulsing of vaginal muscles.

TIME/REPS: Hold bridge for one minute with three Kegels, taking five breaths to hold and five breaths to release the contraction.

1. Lie on your back with your knees bent and your feet placed hip distance apart, four inches in front of your sitbones.

2. Roll the outer tips of your shoulders under you by lifting your back up slightly and puffing your chest. Slide your shoulder blades down away from your ears and toward each other.

3. Press your feet, shoulder heads, and inner and outer arms evenly into the floor (do not press with the back of your head or neck). Lift your back up, taking your spine deeply into your body and opening your chest.

4. Drop your inner thighs down toward the floor while you move your tailbone up into your body and open your chest more.

5. Bring your awareness to the area of your pelvic floor, including the muscles around your anus, the muscles of the vagina, and the muscles supporting the uterus and intestines.

6. Begin to contract the vaginal/anal muscles (as though you were trying to stop the flow of urine) without tightening your buttock muscles. Start by contracting with each *exhale* and releasing with each *inhale*. Then tighten for five breaths and release for five breaths.

MENTAL FOCUS: Notice the internal sensation of your hips, pelvis, and breath meeting through the fluid sensual movement patterns you are applying to the shape. Focus on keeping your pelvic floor lifted and on pumping your vaginal muscles, contracting them on the *exhale* and releasing them on the *inhale.* As you do this exercise, notice any emotions that arise from the sensation in your hips, pelvis, and buttocks. Use your breath to move these feelings through your body.

BENEFITS: Bridge Series expands your upper torso while strengthening your back, hips, buttocks, and hamstrings, promoting digestion and invigorating your body. By combining Bridge Pose with Kegel pulsing (also known as Mula Bandha, or pelvic floor exercise), this series promotes a stronger libido by creating a greater flow of awareness and circulation throughout the whole pelvic area.

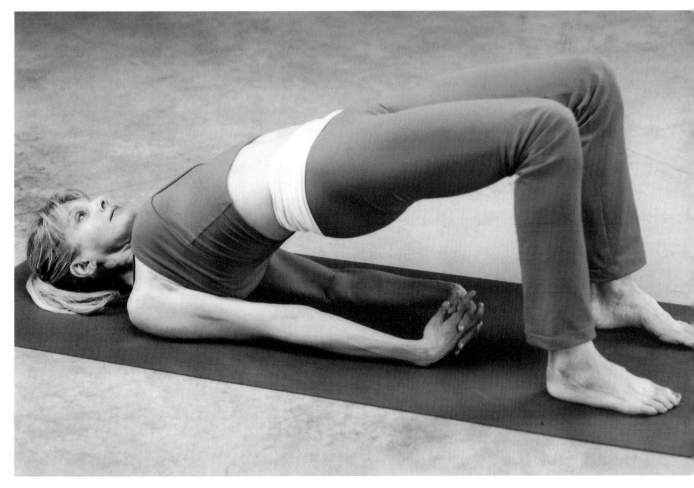

Bridge Pose Series— Pelvic Tilts

MOVEMENT FOCUS: Pelvic tilt.

REPS: Ten, with ten pulses at the top.

1. Starting in the raised Bridge position (page 172), tighten your buttock muscles around your sitbones. Place your arms out to the sides.

2. *With the exhalation,* tilt your pubic bone toward your navel, lifting your whole pelvis toward the sky. Completely scoop the pelvis as you press your navel toward your lower back.

3. *With the inhalation,* lower your spine back to the floor, vertebra by vertebra, and press your sitbones into the floor, tilting your pubic bone toward your tailbone.

4. Once your lower back is down on the floor, keep inhaling and gently lift the middle of your spine up off the floor, expanding your chest. Your feet and shoulders stay grounded on the floor.

5. On the next exhalation, press your middle spine into the floor, tilt your pubic bone toward your navel, and lift your pelvis back up.

6. Tilt your pelvis back and forth, up and down, ten times with each *inhale* and *exhale.*

7. After ten cycles, finish with ten small Kegel contracting pulses at the top.

MENTAL FOCUS: Notice the relationships among your breath, pelvis, and spine as you create a fluid tilting action. Breathe deeply, noticing, without judgment, any thoughts and sensations as they arise.

ADVANCED MODIFICATION: Lift one leg and do five cycles on each side.

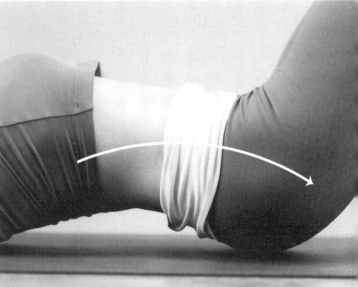

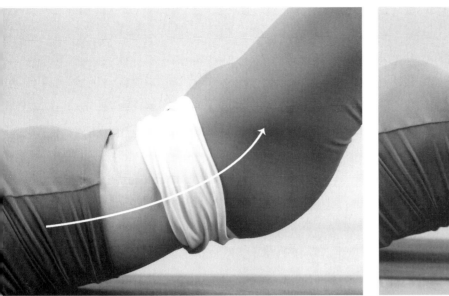

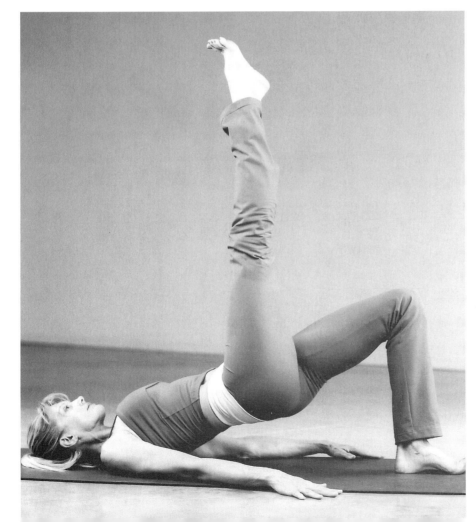

Advanced Modification

Bridge Pose Series— Pelvic Pendulum

Pelvic semicircles side to side.

Ten.

1. Start in raised Bridge position (page 172) with your arms to the sides, and create a semicircular movement side to side in your hips.

2. Keep your shoulder heads and feet pressing into the floor evenly.

3. *Imagine a pendulum swinging:* As your hips swing to the right, your left hip drops; as your hips swing to the left, your right hip drops.

4. Keep the muscles firm around your sitbones and synchronize your movement with your breath.

5. Relax your facial muscles.

MENTAL FOCUS: *Imagine you're sliding your lower back across the inside of a bowl.*

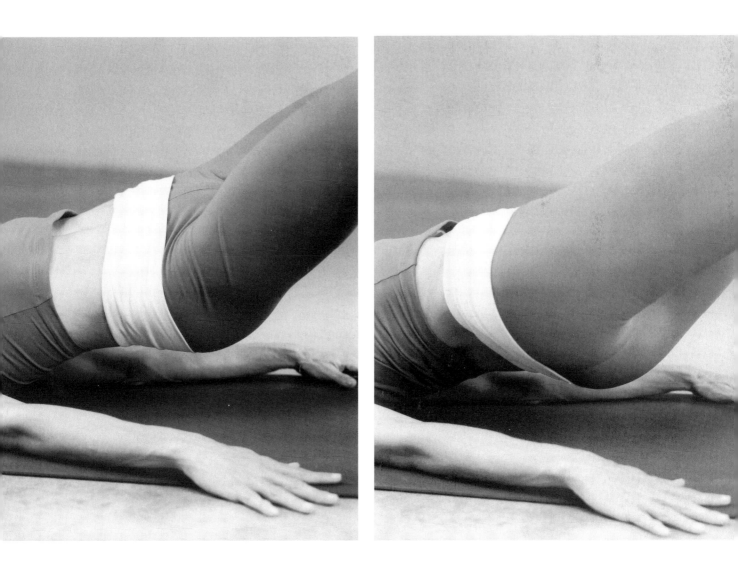

Bridge Pose Series— Circle Dance

MOVEMENT FOCUS: Circles with hips and pelvis.

TIME/REPS: Ten in each direction.

1. Start in raised Bridge position (page 172) with your arms out to the sides.

2. Keep your shoulder heads and feet pressing into the floor evenly.

3. Trace an *entire* circle with your hips. As you make the bottom part of the circle, bring your lower back close to the floor without touching it.

4. Keep your buttock muscles firm around your sitbones as you synchronize your movement with your breath. Try to keep your movement smooth.

5. Relax your jaw and breathe deeply.

ADVANCED MODIFICATION:

1. Lie down on your back and place your heels hip distance apart on the edge of a chair seat.

2. Tilt your pelvis up off the floor as you root your shoulders and inner and outer arms into the floor. Keep your arms out to the sides.

3. Circle your pelvis. As you make the bottom part of the circle, your lower back should come close to the floor without touching it.

MENTAL FOCUS: Enjoy the sensation of your hips swaying and dancing. *Imagine that you are painting a circle in the air with your tailbone.*

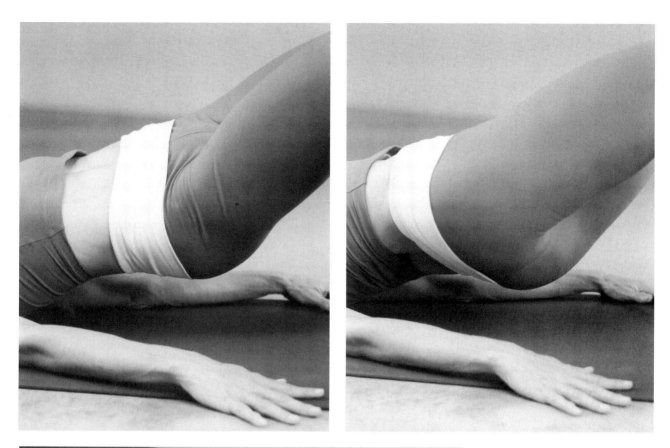

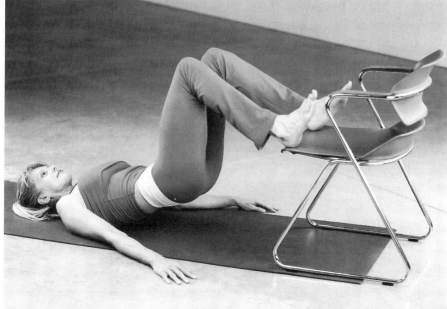

Advanced Modification

Reclining Knees to Chest

MOVEMENT FOCUS: Stillness, organic release, knees drawn to chest.

TIME: Thirty seconds, *inhaling* through your nose, *exhaling* through your mouth.

1. Lie on your back and bring both knees into your chest.

2. *Inhale.* Elongate your entire spine from your tailbone through the crown of your head.

3. *Exhale,* drawing your knees deeper into your chest and pressing your lower back into the floor.

4. Feel the release in your lumbar spine and a gentle firming in your lower abdominal muscles.

5. Take several breaths, *inhaling* through your nose and *exhaling* with a sigh through your mouth.

MENTAL FOCUS: Notice the quality of release as you allow your muscles to unfurl, breathe, and let go. Focus on the nonverbal sensations that arise.

BENEFITS: The benefit of a grounding and releasing pose is that it gives you an opportunity to pause—to release physiologically, to listen inwardly, and to notice what arises in the empty space of stillness.

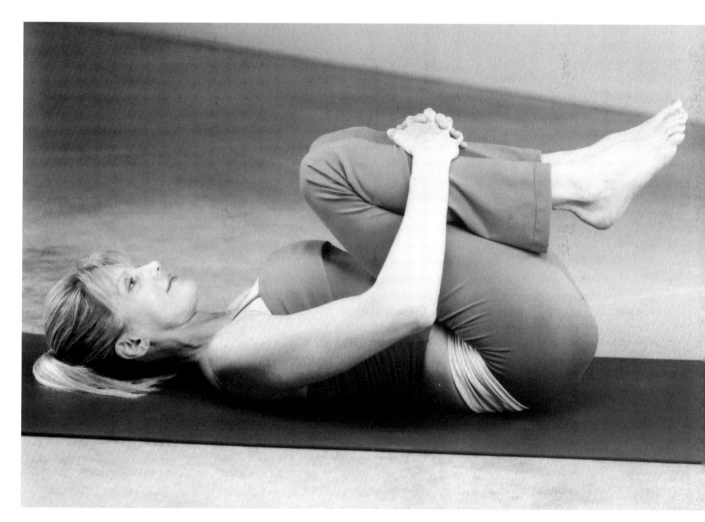

Alligator
Lift

MOVEMENT FOCUS: Expanding energy outward from the core.

REPS: Ten full lifts on each side, plus ten shallow pulses at the top.

1. Roll over onto your left hip and extend your legs, ankles together. (If you have trouble keeping your balance during this exercise, bend your left knee to ninety degrees.)

2. Rest on your left forearm, placing your elbow underneath your left shoulder.

3. Lift your hips up and down six to twelve inches off the floor.

4. Stretch your upper arm up as you lift.

5. Do ten full lifts, then hold at the top and do ten more shallow lifts from that point.

6. Switch sides and repeat.

MENTAL FOCUS: Move from the inside. Use core awareness to lift your body. Move with your breath, noticing how your breath initiates and supports the movement. Keep your face and jaw relaxed.

BENEFITS: Tones and draws awareness to the core, outer thighs, and buttocks.

BEGINNING MODIFICATION: Keep lower leg bent at ninety degrees and keep left hand on the floor for better balance.

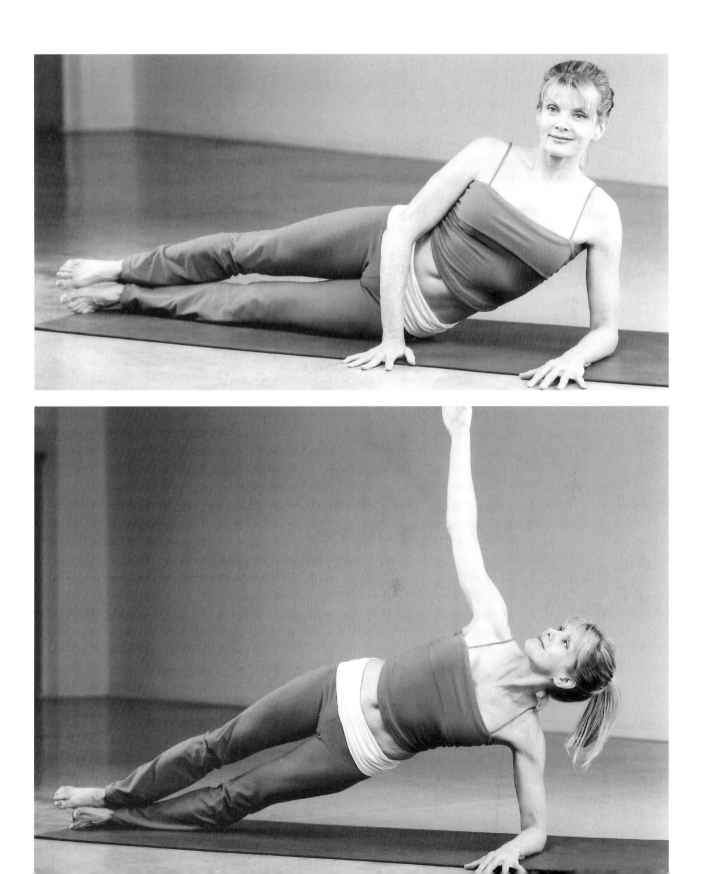

Alligator Dance

Contracting and expanding movement in spine and legs.

Ten on each side—*exhale* as you contract; *inhale* as you expand.

1. Roll over onto your left hip and bend your left leg ninety degrees.

2. Rest on your left forearm, with your elbow underneath your right shoulder.

3. *Exhale,* drawing your right knee into your chest, forehead toward your knee, contracting into a ball as best you can.

4. *Inhale.* Unfurl and straighten your left leg backward.

5. Reach your left arm forward. Stretch your toes and fingertips away from each other.

6. *Exhale* and curl up again.

7. Try to create a smooth, wavelike movement as you contract and expand.

8. Do ten repetitions, switch sides, and repeat.

Speed up the tempo and try exhaling through your mouth as you bring your knee to your chest.

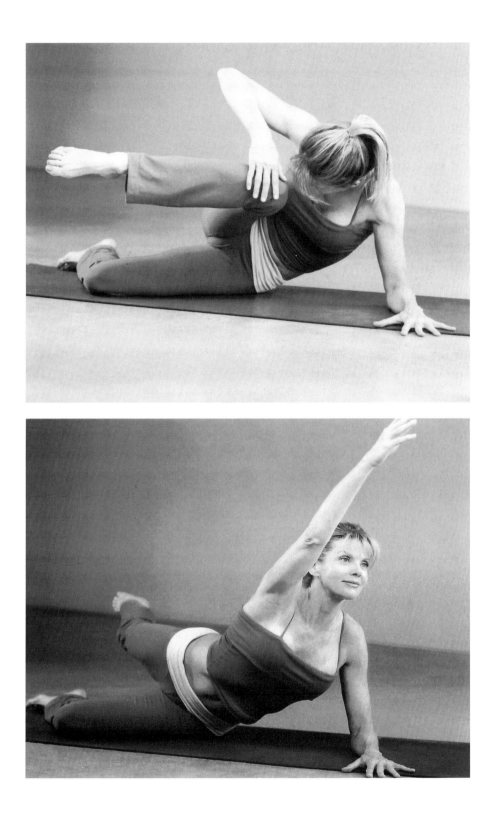

Child's Pose 1

Melting shoulders around knees; stillness.

Thirty seconds.

1. Begin on your hands and knees, with your knees and shins together.

2. Keeping your hands on the floor, sit back, drawing your sitbones toward your heels.

3. Lay your chest onto your thighs, wrapping your shoulders around your knees, and place your forehead on the floor.

4. Place your hands, palms up, by your feet.

5. Allow your breath to stay smooth and your facial and jaw muscles to soften.

6. Relax completely, allowing your forehead, shoulders, belly, and hips to release.

7. With each *inhale,* feel an expansion between your shoulder blades; with each *exhale,* allow your whole body to melt into the Earth.

BENEFITS: Child's Pose relaxes, releases, and grounds all at once. It is a rejuvenating posture that helps us draw our awareness inward in a calm, effortless way.

NOTE: If you have any knee pain, place a bed pillow behind your knees to support them.

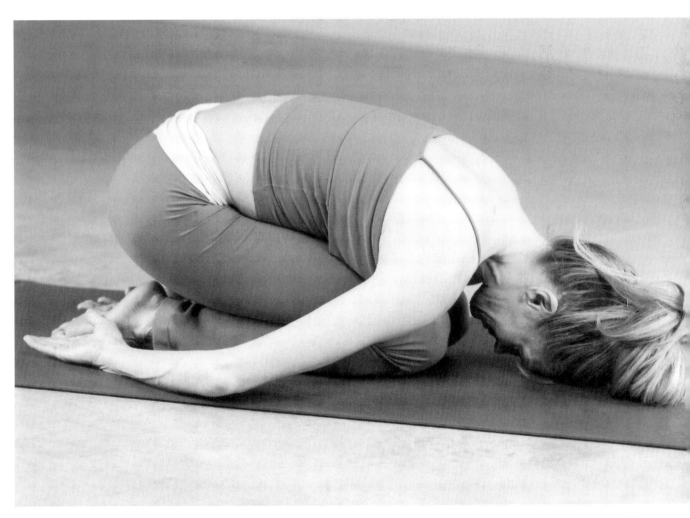

Cat's Breath— Slow

Spine movement like a semicircle flexing slowly up and down.

REPS: Ten, with long breaths through your nose.

1. Start on your hands and knees.

2. Place your hands directly underneath your shoulders, middle finger forward, and knees directly underneath your hips.

3. Establish a smooth, flowing ujjayi breath in the back of your throat.

4. Create a line of energy in each arm by pressing down, elongating your arms. Elongate your spine from your tailbone to the crown of your head.

5. *Exhale,* tucking your hips and rounding your back into a Cat Tilt. Firm your buttocks and draw in your stomach as you draw your tailbone and forehead toward each other.

6. *Inhale,* soften your belly, and lift your head, chest, and tailbone upward, creating the Dog Tilt as you spill the top of your pelvis forward and arch your back.

7. Keep pressing down into your arms, lifting out of your shoulders as you open your chest.

8. Create a smooth arching curve in your lower back as you continue to draw your navel toward your spine and reach your sitbones upward.

9. Gently rock back and forth between Cat and Dog Tilts. Try to keep a seamless transition between the two movements to begin to create a smooth wave of movement in your spine.

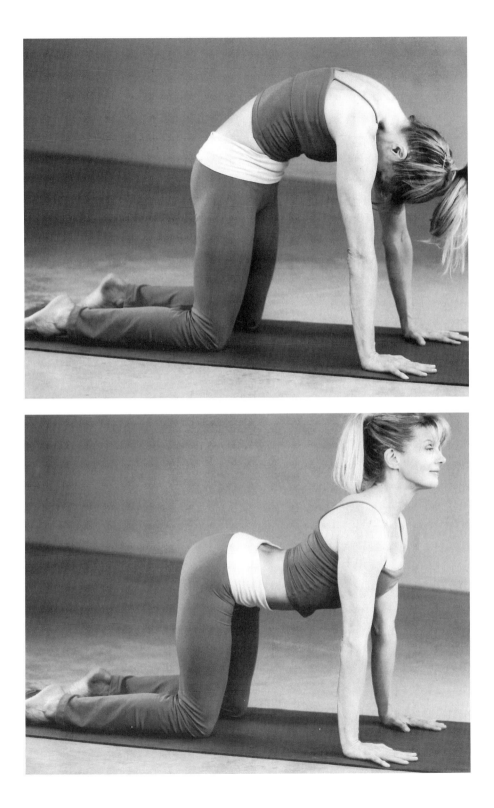

Cat's Breath— Fast

MOVEMENT FOCUS: Semicircle and wave undulation in spine.

REPS: Fifteen fast with breaths, *inhaling* through your nose, *exhaling* through your mouth.

1. Begin as in Cat's Breath—Slow (page 188).

2. Speed up the rhythm of your breath and movement, *inhaling* through your nose as you lift your head, chest, and sitbones.

3. *Exhale* through your mouth as you round your back.

4. Synchronize your breath and movement so that each part of your movement is driven by the inhale or exhale.

5. Keep your neck fluid but supported, not overly loose.

6. Smooth out the transition between the two positions to create a fluid quality to your movement.

7. If you feel dizzy from the rapid breathing, rest in Child's Pose 1 (page 186) for a few moments before continuing to the next exercise.

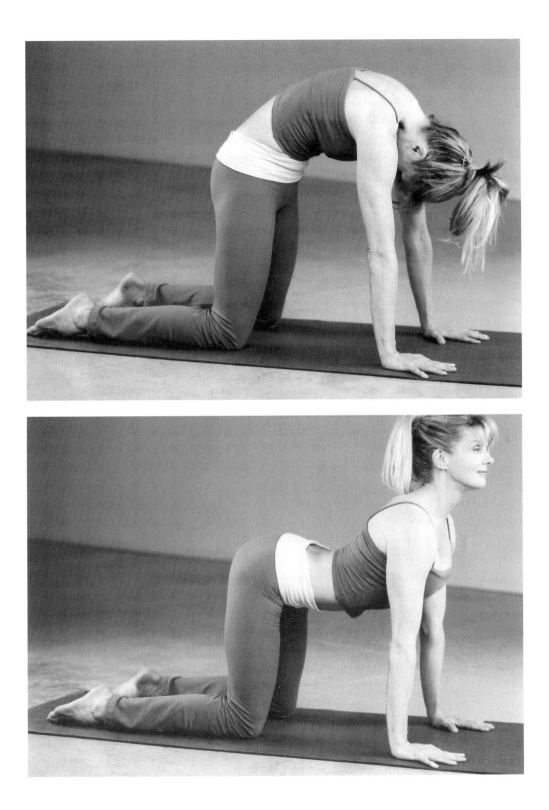

Cat's Breath— Knee to Chest

MOVEMENT FOCUS: Draw your knee closer to your chest on each exhale as your spine rounds.

TIME: Thirty seconds on each leg.

1. Place your hands under your shoulders, and your left knee directly under your left hip.

2. Create a Cat Tilt, rounding your spine as you draw your right knee into your chest. Lift the foot off the floor as your forehead and knee reach toward each other.

3. Bring your knee as close to your chest as possible for thirty seconds on each side. Keep your breathing steady.

4. Be mindful to keep your organs of perception (eyes, lips, tongue, jaw) relaxed.

5. Focus on firming your buttocks around your sitbones.

6. Keep your arms elongated, rooting down through both hands and your bottom shin to stabilize the pose.

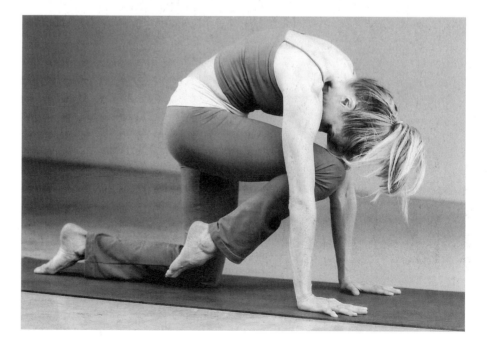

MOVEMENT FOCUS: The inner spiral of your thigh lifts toward the sky as your knee lifts.

TIME: Thirty seconds on each leg.

1. Place both hands under your shoulders, and your left knee directly under your left hip. Create a Dog Tilt by arching your back.

2. Firm your buttocks, ground your left sitbone toward the Earth, and lift your right leg at a ninety-degree angle toward the sky. Flex your right foot and spread its toes.

3. Create an inner spiral of energy in the lifted leg, rolling your inner thigh toward the ceiling. Keep your hips level.

4. Pull your navel toward your spine to protect your lower back.

5. Stay attentive to the steadiness of your breath as you keep your leg lifted for thirty seconds on each side.

Cat's Breath— Knee to Sky

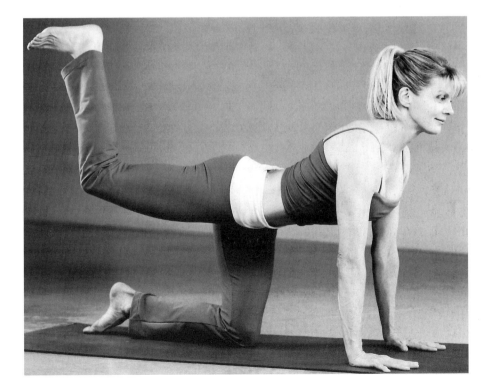

Hips, Pelvis, and Legs

Cat's Breath— Knee Dance 1

Semicircle and wave undulation in spine.

Ten on each leg, plus ten pulses at the top.

1. Keep both hands placed under your shoulders, your left knee under your left hip.

2. *Exhale* as you draw your right knee into your chest, forehead toward your knee.

3. *Inhale,* arch your back to create a Dog Tilt, and extend your right leg up.

4. Move back and forth between the two shapes, using your breath and creating a fluid, rhythmic wavelike movement in your spine.

5. *Inhale* as you look up and elongate through the back of your neck.

6. *Exhale* completely, as you look to your knees and round your spine.

7. Move back and forth for ten cycles on each leg, focusing on keeping your buttocks firm the whole time.

8. After ten cycles, hold the Dog Tilt and pulse your lifted leg ten times, lifting and lowering your knee in one-inch pulses.

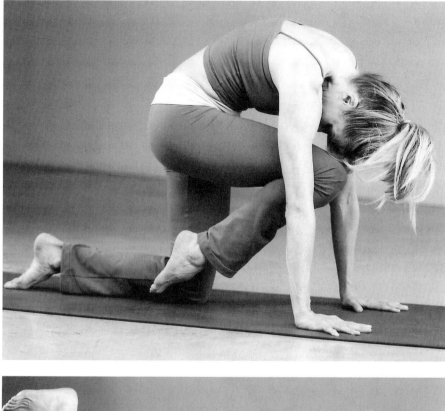

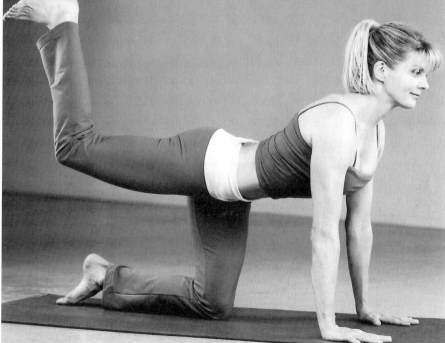

Cat's Breath— Knee Dance 2

MOVEMENT FOCUS: Circles with femur and knee; neutral spine.

REPS: Twenty circles with each leg.

1. Keep both hands placed under your shoulders, your left knee under your left hip.

2. Make a circle with your right knee, keeping your spine and pelvis neutral and still.

3. Protect your lower back by drawing your navel toward your spine and your left sitbone toward the Earth.

4. Make twenty big circles with your right knee bent, heel toward your buttock.

5. Draw as big a circle as you can while keeping your spine and pelvis as still as possible.

6. Focus on opening up the full range of movement in your hip joint, isolating the thigh bone from the hip joint. Enjoy the sensation of your hips and buttocks heating up. Relax your facial muscles and neck.

7. Move at a pace that allows you to breathe steadily and maintain fluid movements.

MENTAL FOCUS: What feelings arise as you begin to energize and empower your hips, pelvis, and legs?

ADVANCED MODIFICATION: Combine this movement with Slow Cat's Breath (page 188) movement in your spine, keeping your navel in, creating an undulating spine along with the circling action of your knee. Focus on keeping your neck relaxed.

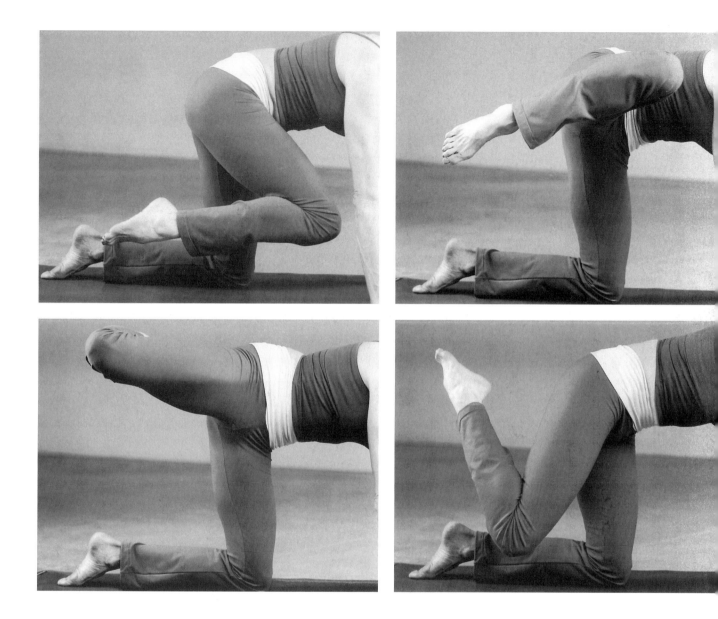

Uttanasana

Stillness; legs ground as shoulder blades move into the back.

Thirty seconds.

1. Stand with your feet parallel, hip distance apart, and root your feet down into the Earth.

2. Interlace your fingers behind your back.

3. *Inhale* as you roll your shoulders down away from your ears and draw your shoulder blades toward each other.

4. *Exhale* and fold forward, taking your arms up and over while keeping your shoulders lifted away from your ears.

5. Keep your thighs lifted and feel into the release of your shoulders, back muscles, and hamstrings.

BENEFITS: Uttanasana will help release and open your back body and shoulders.

NOTE: Do not lock your knees. If your hamstrings are tight or strained, bend your knees slightly.

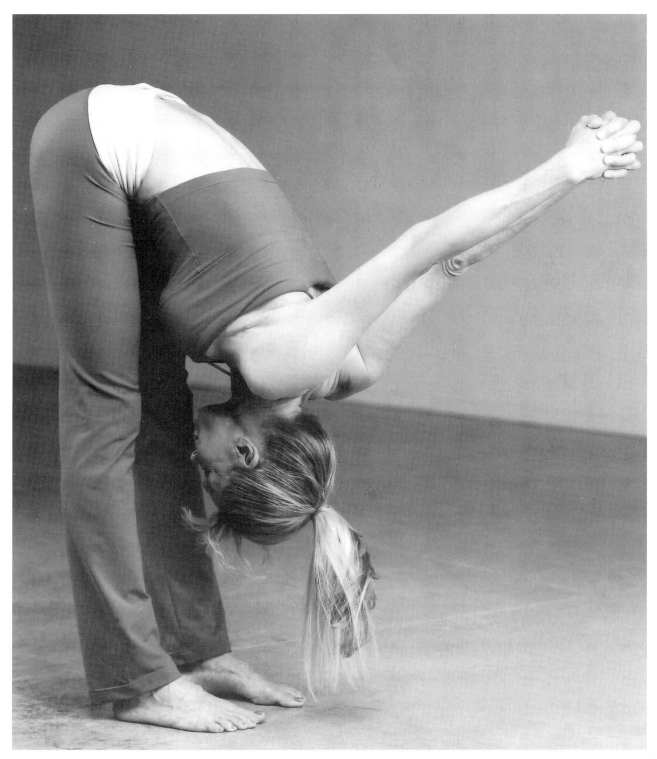

Chair— Root

Stillness; elongation of spine.

One minute, pulsing one inch up and down for the last fifteen seconds.

1. Stand with your feet together. Place your palms together, arms overhead.

2. Bend your knees, pressing the front of your knees toward the back of your heels.

3. As you move into a seated posture, elongate your spine diagonally upward through the crown of your head.

4. Take deep and steady breaths.

5. Keep your shoulders relaxed and away from your ears; keep your eyes and jaw soft.

MENTAL FOCUS: *Imagine your legs steady and firm like a tree trunk; your arms and spine stretching upward and outward, flexible, like branches blowing in the wind.*

BENEFITS: Chair Pose Series will help you cultivate fluid strength in your entire lower torso. This series will also enable you to integrate the rooting strength of the lower torso with the uplifting fluidity of the upper torso.

MODIFICATION: Hook your thumbs together, spreading your other fingers apart, and take your hands overhead. Pull outward and down with your arms to create space around your neck as you continue to elongate through your torso.

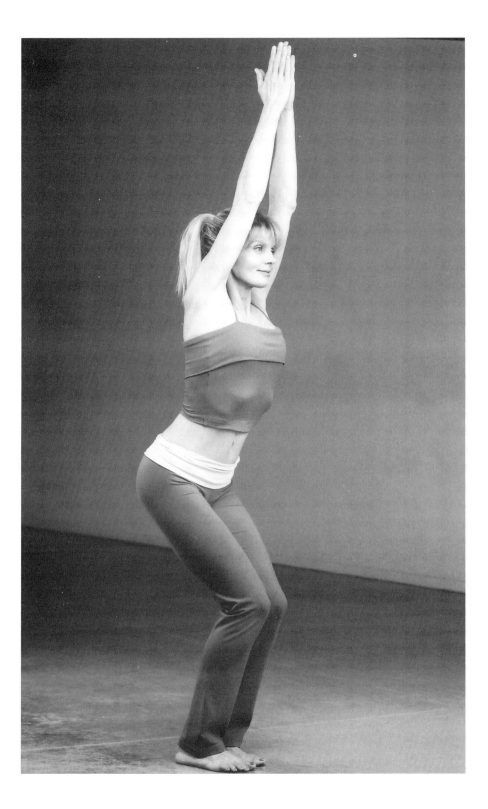

Chair— Root Dance

Sagittal wave motion from roots through spine.

Eight.

1. Stand with your feet hip distance apart for extra stability.

2. *Exhale,* sweeping your arms forward and folding forward over your bent legs, releasing your spine and head with the breath.

3. Lay your ribs over your thighs as you sweep your arms down behind your back. As your arms reach the limit of their range, straighten your knees and stretch your arms up.

4. *Inhale,* swinging your arms forward again and elongating your spine. Lift your ribs off your thighs, letting the momentum carry you into a slight backward stretch.

5. Repeat eight times. Enjoy the wave of movement that flows from your *roots*—your foundation in your legs—all the way up your spine and back with each inhale and exhale.

6. Feel how breath and momentum work together to create movement in your core.

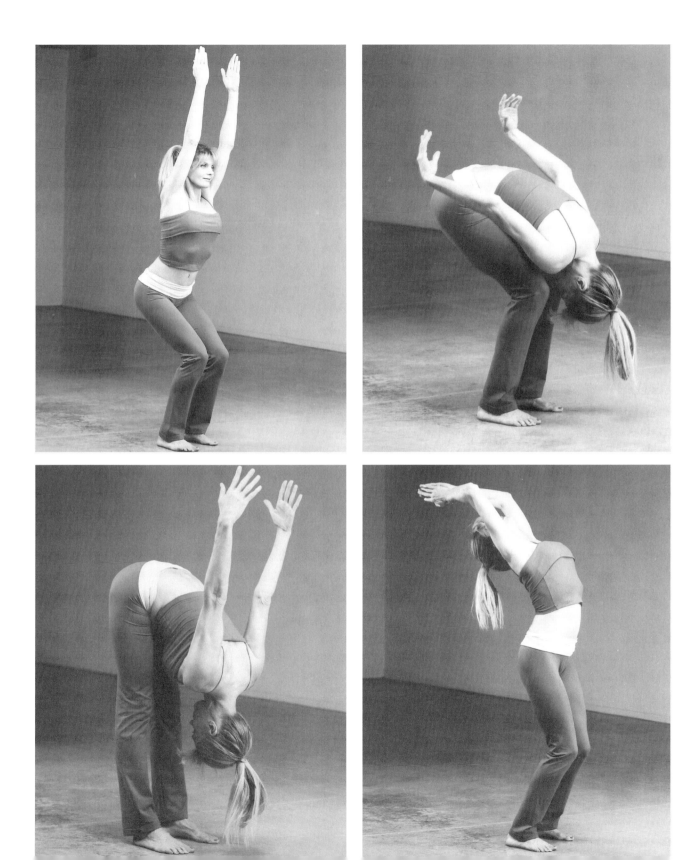

Chair—
Hip Dance

1. Start in Chair—Root (page 200) with your big toes, inner ankles, and inner knees touching.

2. Stretch your arms out wide like wings, reaching out through the middle finger of each hand. Keep your shoulders down away from your ears.

3. Circle your hips ten times to the right and then ten times to the left.

4. Feel your hips tracing a complete horizontal circle.

5. Keep all four corners of your feet rooted into the floor and enjoy the feeling of connection to the Earth.

6. Keep your knees bent and see if you can create a spiral of movement traveling up from your hips, like a vine, all the way up through the crown of your head and out through each finger!

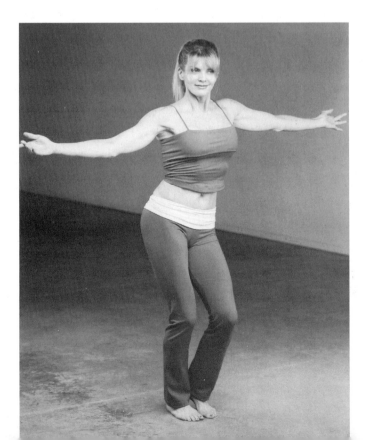

MOVEMENT FOCUS: Circles in hips, knees, and metatarsals.

REPS: Ten circles in each direction.

1. Start in Chair—Root (page 200) with your big toes, inner ankles, and inner knees touching.

2. Place one hand on each knee and reach your sitbones toward your heels as if you were sitting down into a chair.

3. Keep your knees together and make ten complete circles in each direction with your knees touching.

4. Move your weight to the front of your feet as your knees come to the front of the circle. Take your weight back into your heels as your knees trace the back side of the circle.

BENEFITS: This helps safely condition and lubricate the connective tissue in the knees.

Chair— Hip/Knee Dance

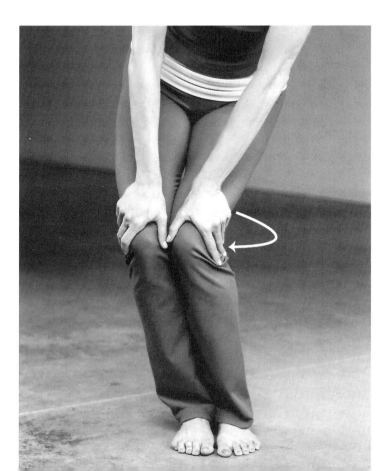

Uttanasana with Arms Wrapped Behind Calves

MOVEMENT FOCUS: Stillness; back expands between shoulder blades.

TIME: Thirty seconds.

1. Stand with your feet slightly less than hip distance apart.

2. Taking your arms behind you, bring your hands between your legs and grasp opposing shins.

3. Root your feet down into the Earth and make your legs firm.

4. Round up toward the sky through the space between your shoulder blades.

5. Focus on keeping your back rounded to release the muscles along your spine.

6. Expand your ribs on each *inhale.*

7. Keep your thighs lifted and feel into the release of your shoulders, back muscles, and hamstrings.

BENEFITS: Uttanasana will help release and open your back body and shoulders.

BEGINNING MODIFICATION: Place your hands or elbows on your thighs and keep your knees slightly bent.

NOTE: Do not lock your knees. If your hamstrings are tight or strained, bend your knees slightly.

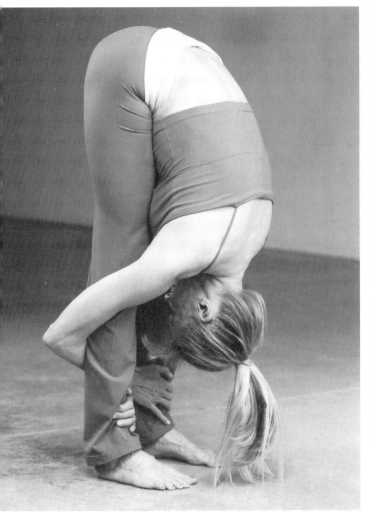 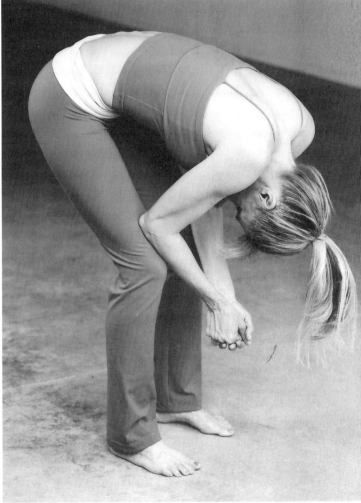

Beginning Modification

Door
Dance 1

Pelvic tilts; spinal flexion.

REPS: Eight pelvic tilts—*inhale* chest open, *exhale* round back.

1. Taking hold of the knobs on either side of an open door, place your feet hip distance apart and about a foot and a half away from the door.

2. Come onto the ball of each foot, lifting your heels off the floor.

3. Make sure your knees are directly over your ankles.

4. Elongate your arms, leaning your weight back away from the door.

5. Bend your knees until your thighs are parallel to the floor.

6. *Inhale,* spilling your pelvis forward and opening your chest (as in a Dog Tilt).

7. *Exhale* completely, reversing your pelvic tilt, pulling your pubic bone up toward your navel and rounding your back.

8. Stay on the balls of your feet; keep your thighs parallel to the floor and your arms extended.

MENTAL FOCUS: As you continue to explore the power of fluid, circular movement in your hips, notice an even greater awakening of vital energy in your pelvis, hips, and legs.

BENEFITS: Door Dance Series will help you cultivate fluid strength in your entire lower torso. Using the door helps stabilize your spine and core and isolate movement in your hip joints.

NOTE: Be sure to use a door with sturdy hinges and knobs.

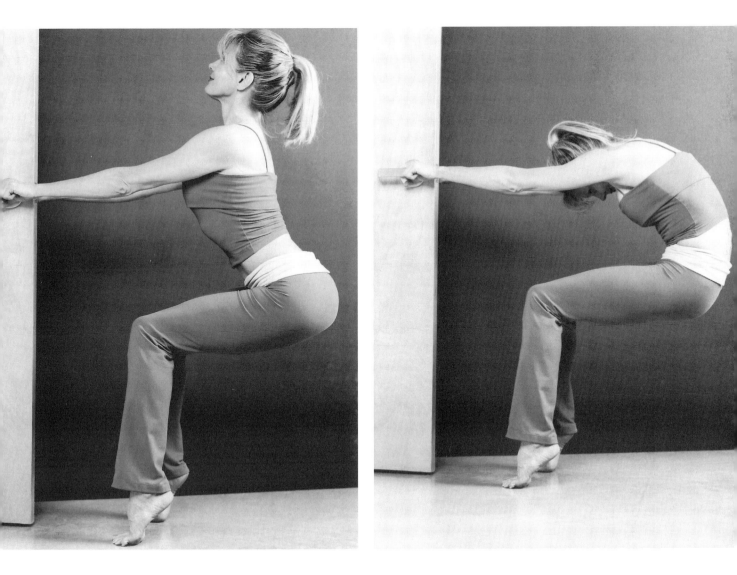

Door
Release—
Squat

MOVEMENT FOCUS: Stillness.

TIME: Thirty seconds.

1. Begin as in Door Dance 1 (page 208).

2. Keeping your hands on the doorknobs, bend your knees out to the sides and come into a full yogic squat.

3. Feel into the release of your back muscles as well as the opening of your hips.

4. Make sure that you are far enough away from the edge of the door to get a full stretch in your arms and back.

5. Keep your chin in. *Breathe* smoothly and steadily.

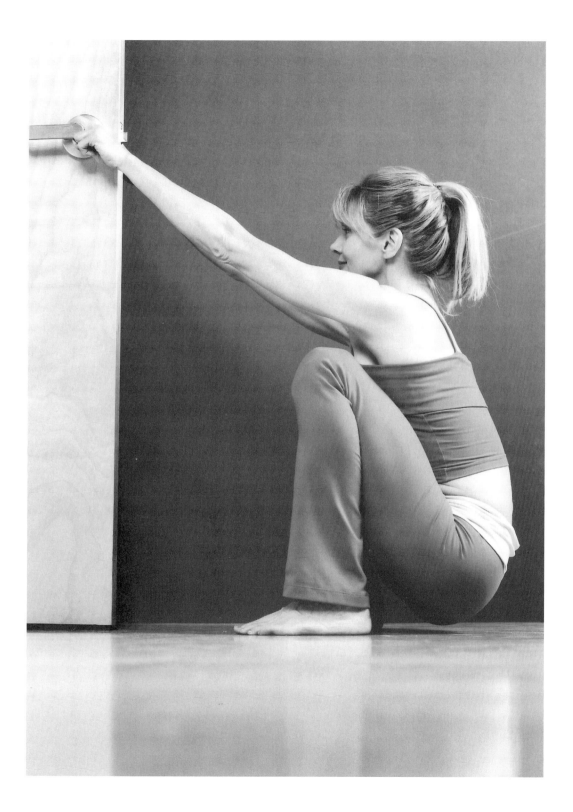

Temple Squat— Hold

REPS: Ten breaths, plus ten pulses.

1. Place your feet three and a half to four feet apart and turn them out slightly (not more than forty-five degrees). Bend your knees, lowering your sitbones until your thighs come parallel to the Earth.

2. Draw up your inner arches as you root down into the Earth through all four corners of each foot.

3. Press your outer knees toward your little toes, keeping your knees stacked over your ankles. *Do not let your ankles collapse inward.*

4. Keep your spine perpendicular to the ground.

5. Now firm, firm, firm your buttocks around your sitbones and feel your whole lower torso awaken.

6. Place one hand on the top of each knee and let your shoulders ride up toward your ears.

7. Elongate the entire spine and both right and left sides of your rib cage as you sink your sitbones deeper toward the Earth. Stop sinking when your thighs are parallel to the floor.

8. Take ten breaths, then do ten one-inch pulses up and down.

MENTAL FOCUS: *Imagine your legs sucking energy up from the Earth just as a plant drinks from its roots.* This stance is First Position in all West African dances and serves as a way to connect the dancer's body to the power of the Earth. Celebrate the power and beauty of your hips.

BENEFITS: Like the Door Dance Series, the Temple Squat Series will cultivate fluid strength in your entire lower torso through a powerful spiral action in the hips. You may notice a quivering in your legs as you build the stamina of your root, or supporting, system. Focus on creating circular, flowing patterns of movement in your hips and spine as energy moves upward from your feet. Keep your face soft and relaxed and enjoy the dance!

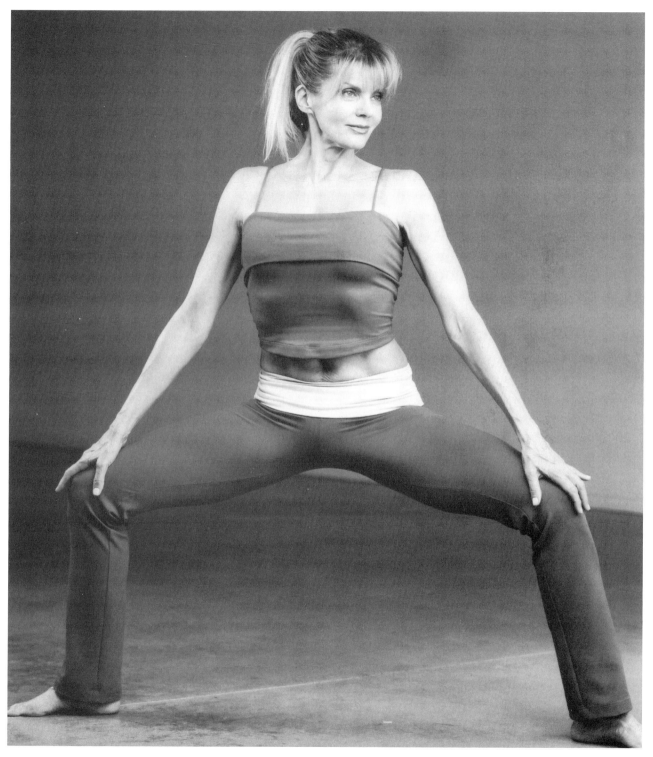

Temple Squat— Twist

MOVEMENT FOCUS: Stillness, rooting action in legs, spiral in spine.

REPS: Eight on each side.

1. Place your feet three and a half to four feet apart and turn them out slightly (no more than forty-five degrees). Bend your knees, lowering your sitbones until your thighs come parallel to the Earth.

2. Draw up your inner arches as you root down into the Earth through all four corners of each foot.

3. Press your outer knees toward your little toes, keeping your knees stacked over your ankles. *Do not let your ankles collapse inward.*

4. Keep your spine perpendicular to the ground.

5. Now firm, firm, firm your buttocks around your sitbones and feel your whole lower torso awaken.

6. Place one hand on the top of each knee.

7. *Inhale* and elongate your spine; *exhale* and twist toward the right, looking over your right shoulder. Keep both arms atraight.

8. Enjoy the feeling of opening in your spine as your lower torso continues to yield to the Earth.

9. *Inhale* back to the center. *Exhale* as you twist to the other side.

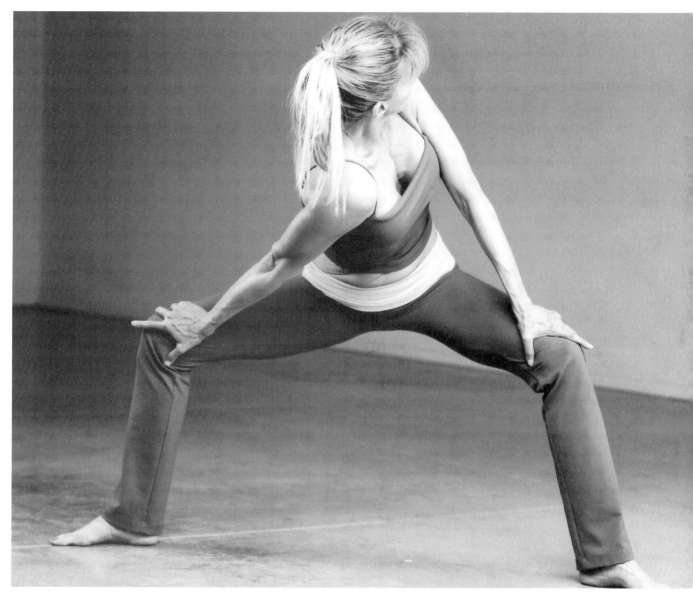

Temple Squat— Hip Dance

MOVEMENT FOCUS: Circles in hips.

REPS: Ten circles in each direction with your hands to your head; ten circles in each direction with your hands on your hips.

1. Place your feet three and a half to four feet apart and turn them out slightly (no more than forty-five degrees). Bend your knees, lowering your pelvis toward the Earth.

2. Draw up your inner arches as you root down into the Earth through all four corners of each foot.

3. Press your outer knees toward your little toes, keeping your knees stacked over your ankles. *Do not let your ankles collapse inward.*

4. Keep your spine perpendicular to the ground.

5. Place your hands on your waist and keep your knees bent.

6. Trace a circle with your hips, rotating your pelvis clockwise ten times. Repeat the circles ten more times in each direction with your hands on your hips.

MENTAL FOCUS: Enjoy the way in which the rotation of the pelvis generates a revitalizing Shakti (feminine life force) within you. Can you allow the powerful movement of your hips to spiral up your spine and into your heart and shoulders?

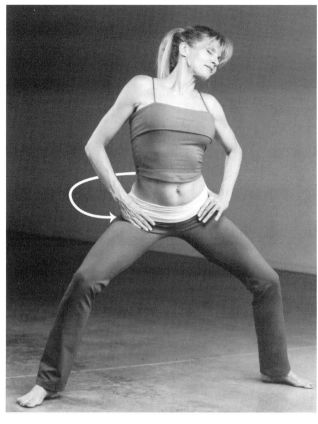
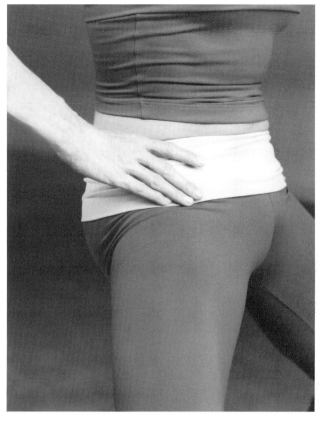
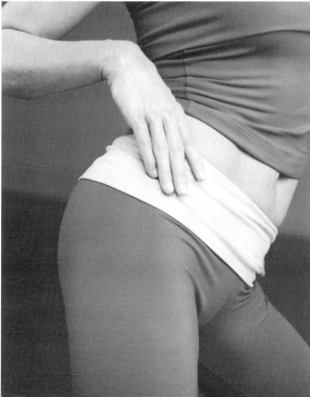
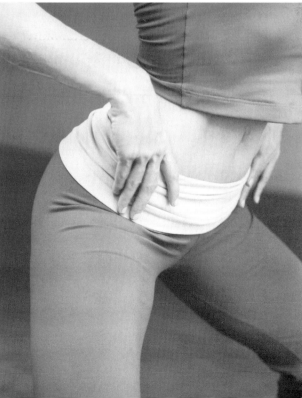

Prasarita Padottana-sana

MOVEMENT FOCUS: Stillness; back body and spine releases.

TIME: Thirty seconds to one minute.

1. Stand with your feet parallel, four feet apart.

2. Fold forward and place your palms on the floor, shoulder distance apart, lining up your fingertips and toes.

3. Draw your elbows toward each other until your forearms come parallel.

4. Keep your shoulders pulled back away from your ears; lift your thighs, keeping your legs firm and the inner arches of your feet lifted.

5. Enjoy the release along the entire back side of your body.

6. Hold for thirty seconds.

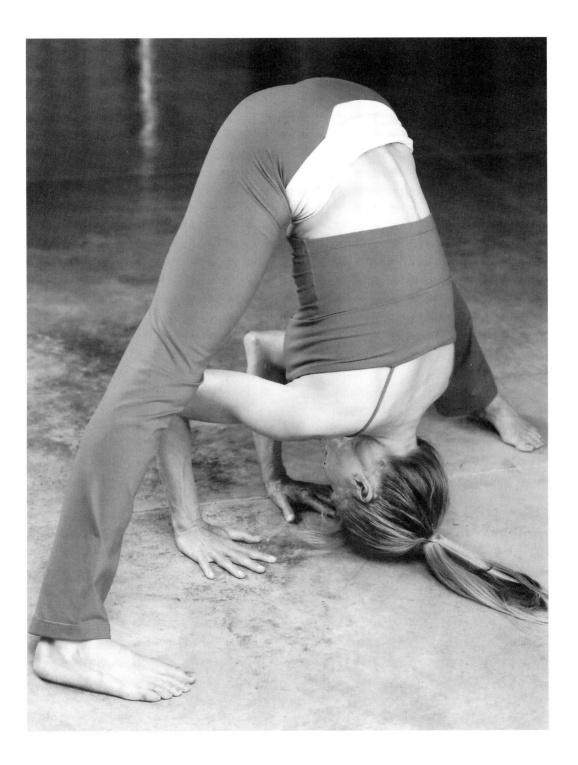

Standing Dance— Foot Circles

MOVEMENT FOCUS: Circles in metatarsals; movement traveling up body.

REPS: Ten fast circles and five slow circles with each leg.

1. Stand with your feet hip distance apart and shift your weight onto your left leg.

2. Lift your right heel and rotate your right foot in circles on the floor.

3. As your right foot circles around the ball of the foot, let the spiral of movement travel up your legs to your hips and all the way up to your shoulders.

4. Switch sides and repeat.

MENTAL FOCUS: Can you create a continuous line of movement between your rotating foot and your shoulders? Following your breath will help you coordinate the movements of your body into a smooth continuum of moving sensation. Enjoy and have fun.

BENEFITS: The Standing Dances in this series will help create an experience of awakening, power, balance, and well-being. They will get your juices flowing while unblocking stuck energy and inhibitions.

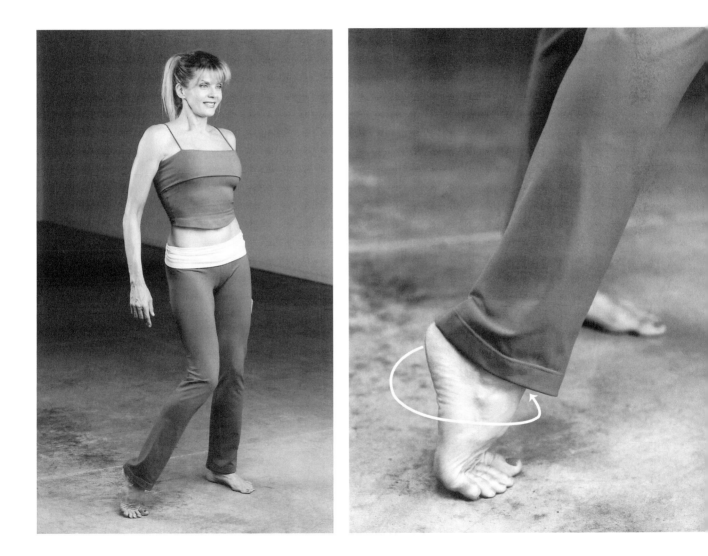

Standing Dance— Hip Circles

MOVEMENT FOCUS: Circles in hips; movement traveling up body.

TIME: One to two minutes on each side.

1. Stand with your feet hip distance apart, or a little wider.

2. Shift your weight onto your left leg without locking the knee.

3. Bend your right knee, lifting your right heel up away from the floor. (This is a similar stance to Standing Dance—Foot Circles (page 220).

4. Trace a circle movement in your hips.

5. Close your eyes and allow your whole body to respond to the circular rhythm of your hips.

6. Switch legs and continue on the other side.

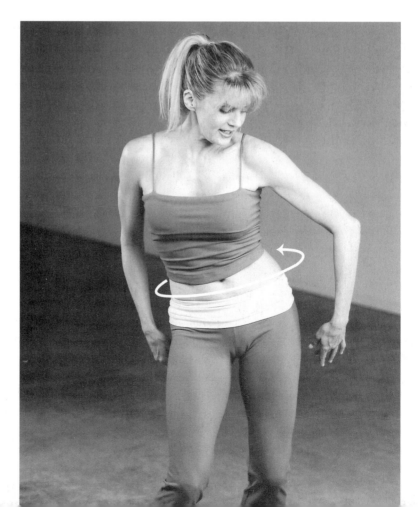

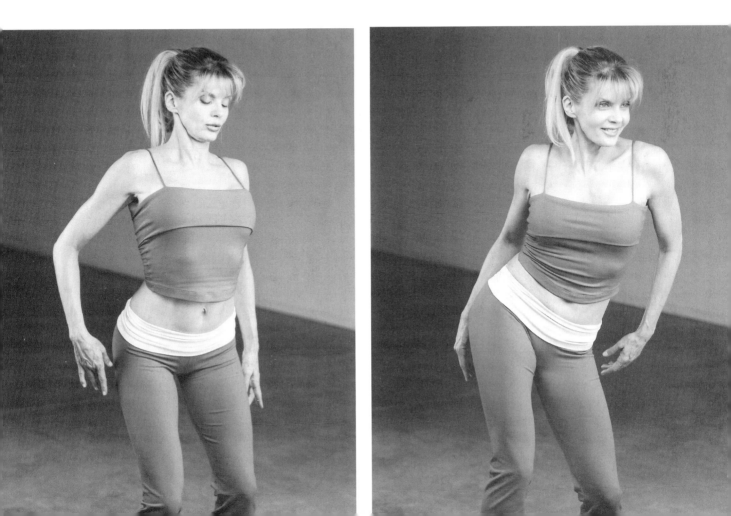

Standing Dance— Figure-8

Figure-8 in hips; movement traveling through limbs.

One to two minutes on each side.

1. Stand with your feet hip distance apart, or a little wider.

2. To make the figure-8, shift your weight back and forth from one foot to the other as you create a circle (half of the figure-8) with one hip at a time.

3. Close your eyes and allow your whole body to respond to the rhythm of your hips.

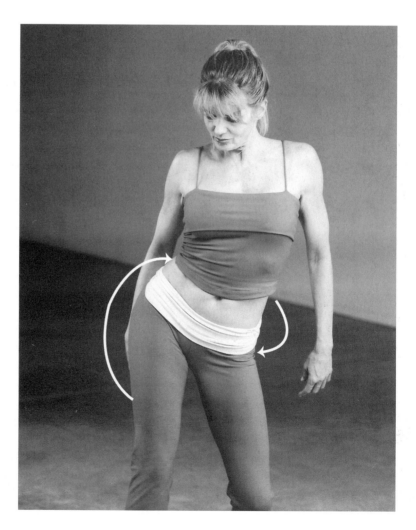

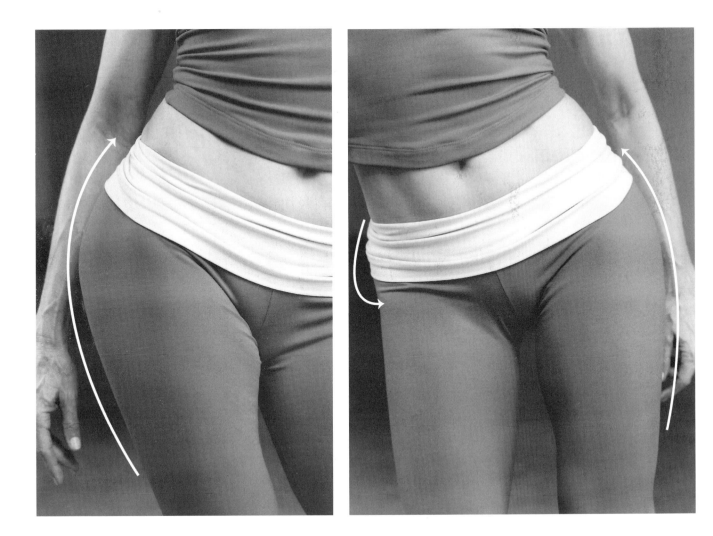

Low Lunge

MOVEMENT FOCUS: Stillness.

TIME: Thirty seconds on each side.

1. Starting on your hands and knees, bring your right foot forward between your hands until the front knee is stacked directly over the ankle.

2. Place extra padding under your back knee.

3. Root down through all four corners of your front foot.

4. Draw your tailbone down into your front body and gently lift your lower belly toward your spine.

5. Feel the release of your hips, left quadriceps, and right hamstring muscles.

6. Your hands may remain on the floor to support the weight of your upper torso, or you can interlace them on top of your front knee.

7. Allow your neck to relax and elongate evenly as you draw your awareness inward.

8. Hold for thirty seconds; switch sides and repeat.

BENEFITS: Releases and opens the hips and stretches the large-muscle groups of the legs and lower back. Stimulates the parasympathetic nervous system (the relaxation response). Helps bring the routine to a calm, meditative close.

ADVANCED MODIFICATION: You can increase the stretch dramatically by placing your back knee and shin against a wall. Make sure your back knee has extra padding, and keep your shin perpendicular to the floor.

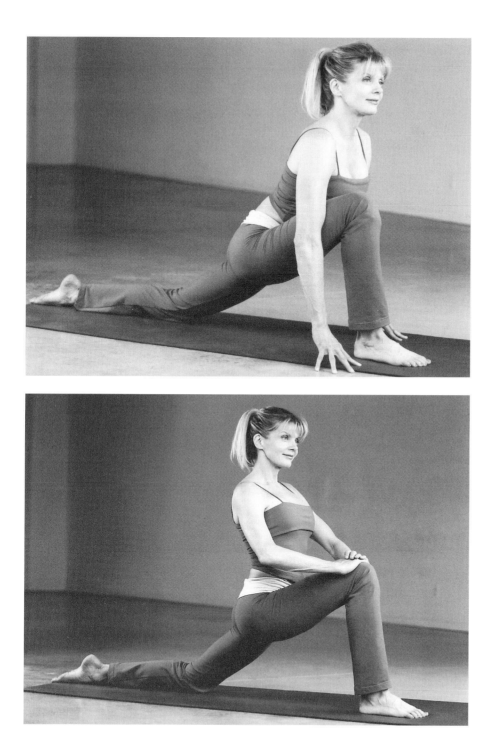

continued on next page

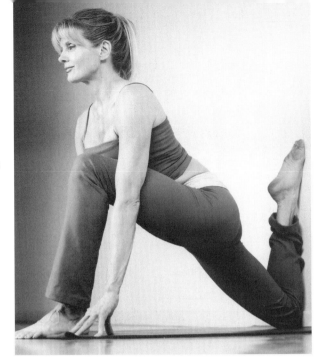

Advanced Modification

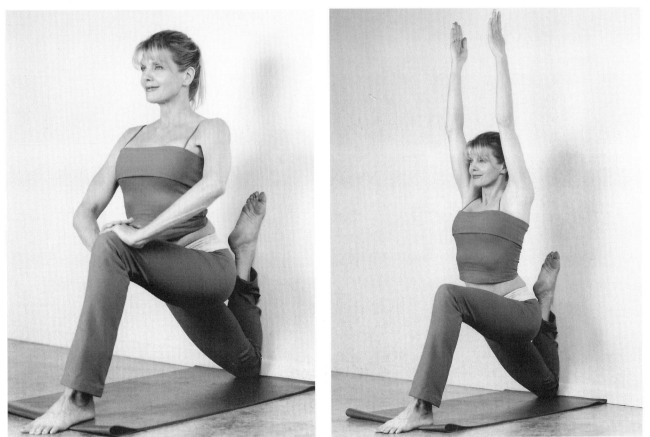

TIME: One minute on each side.

1. Lie down with your sitbones as close as possible to a wall, and your legs up the wall.

2. Cross your right ankle over your left thigh, just above the knee.

3. Start to bend your left knee toward your chest, until your foot comes onto the wall and you begin to feel an opening in your hips.

4. Try to keep your lower back on the floor and use your right hand to gently press your inner right knee toward the wall.

5. As you reach the limit of the stretch, breathe deeply for one minute, then switch sides.

Pigeon at Wall

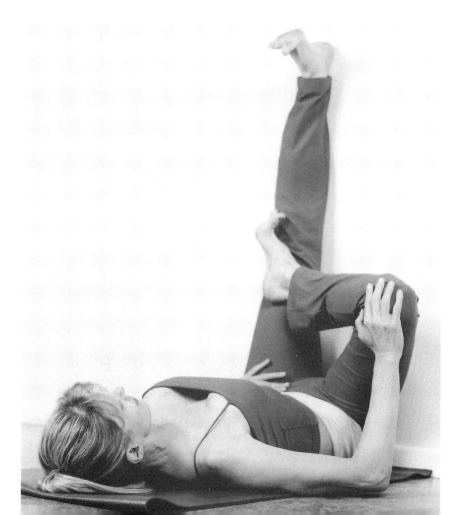

Spinal Twist at Wall

MOVEMENT FOCUS: Stillness.

TIME: One minute on each side.

1. Lie down and take your legs straight up a wall.

2. Draw both knees into your chest.

3. Keeping your inner knees and big toes touching, drop your knees to the right.

4. Your feet should now be on the floor, with the bottoms of your feet still pressing into the wall.

5. Reach out with your left arm and look over your left shoulder.

6. With each *inhale,* elongate your spine.

7. With each *exhale,* deepen the twist.

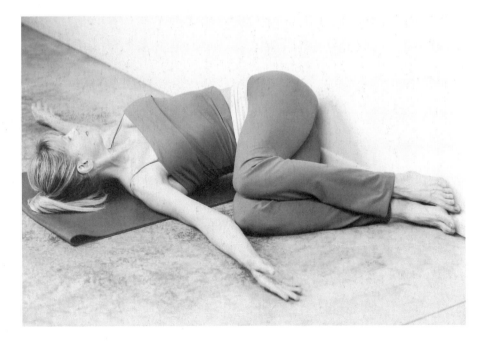

MOVEMENT FOCUS: Stillness.

TIME: One minute.

1. Lie down on your back, with your legs straight up the wall.

2. If possible, have your sitbones touching the wall.

3. Soften your belly and relax your inner groin.

4. Take long, deep breaths.

BENEFITS: This pose is known as the queen of restorative yoga poses. Use it to relax, rejuvenate, and let go.

Viparita Karani

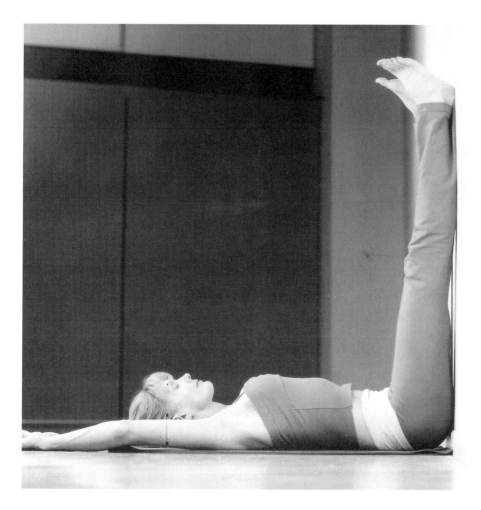

Savasana— Full-Body Meditation

TIME: Three to five minutes.

1. Lie down on your back.

2. Relax your shoulders away from your ears and allow the weight of your bones to surrender to the support of the Earth.

3. Allow a wave of relaxation to wash over you from the top of your head all the way to your toes.

4. Breathe softly and slowly.

5. Soften your face, eyes, lips, tongue, and jaw.

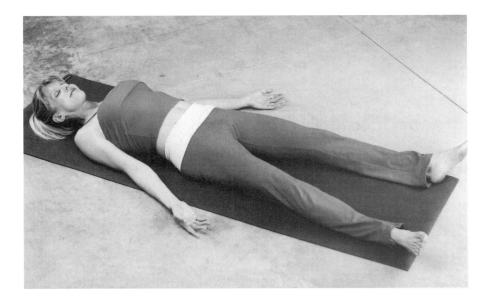

CHAPTER 10

Upper Body

STRONG SHOULDERS, toned arms, and a well-lifted, open chest—these are the physical benefits of training the upper body. At the same time, these physical changes signal an emotional attitude of strength, and openness to the world and to new experiences. You carry so much on your shoulders—it's time to release the pressure, relax, and enjoy the dance!

Mountain Pose

Stillness; internal elongation from Earth to sky.

Thirty seconds.

1. Stand with your big toes and ankles touching.

2. Press down through all four corners of each foot, creating a solid foundation.

3. Firm your thighs.

4. Elongate your spine, reaching upward through the crown of your head.

5. Draw your tailbone into your body as you press your thighs back.

6. Lift your entire rib cage, front and back body, up away from your pelvis.

7. Press your hands together in front of your heart.

8. Bring your focus inward to your center.

BENEFITS: Tones the entire upper torso and increases sensual range of motion of the upper spine, shoulders, arms, and wrists. It will also help release pent-up emotions in your chest.

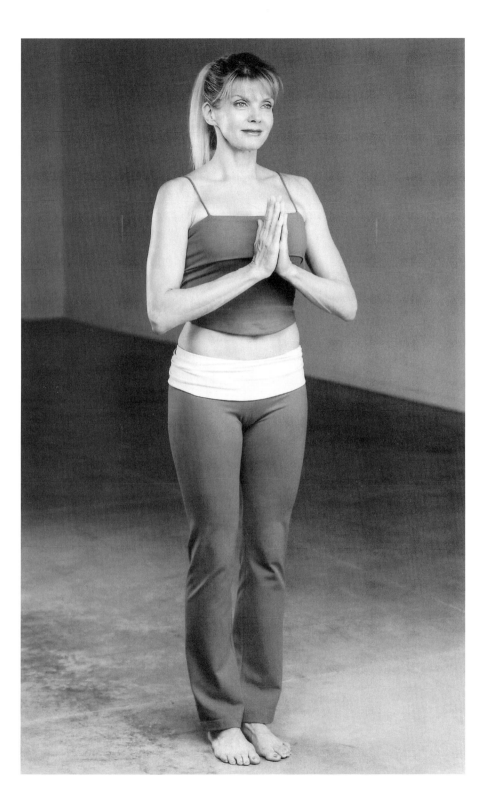

Sunrise Vinyasa

MOVEMENT FOCUS: Meditative movement of arms.

REPS: Three cycles.

1. Begin in Mountain Pose (page 234), with arms down at your sides, palms open.

2. *Inhale* as you reach up, arms outstretched to your sides, touching your palms overhead.

3. *Exhale,* keeping your palms together, and draw your hands down to the center of your chest.

4. Repeat for three cycles.

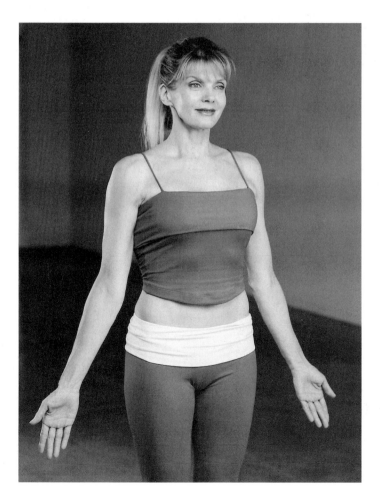

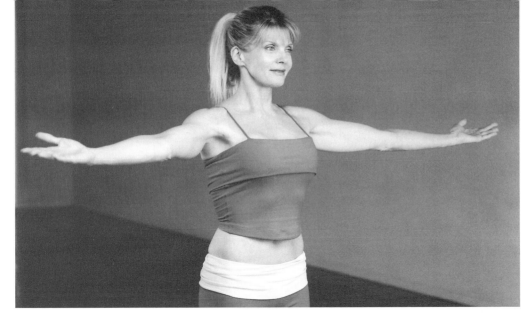

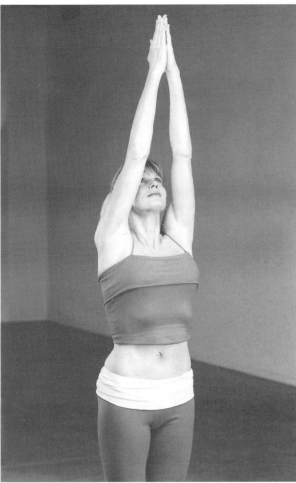

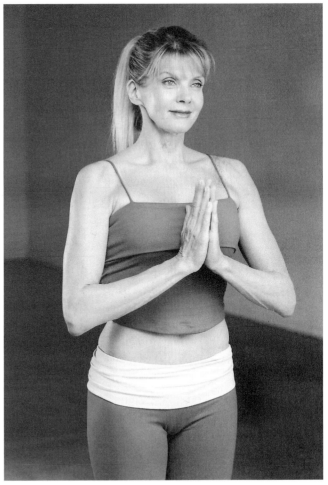

Wrist Circles

Circles in wrists.

Twenty in each direction.

1. Begin in Mountain Pose (page 234).

2. Extend your arms out to each side, parallel to the floor.

3. Keep your arms still and rotate your wrists in complete circles.

4. Focus on extending a line of energy through each arm, from the center of your chest out to your middle finger.

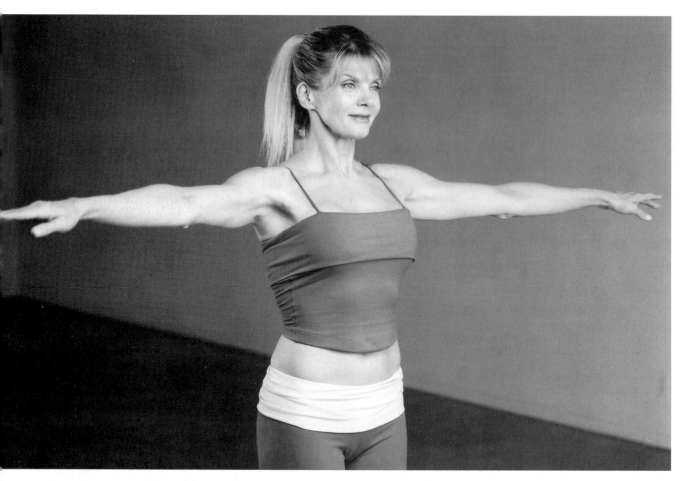

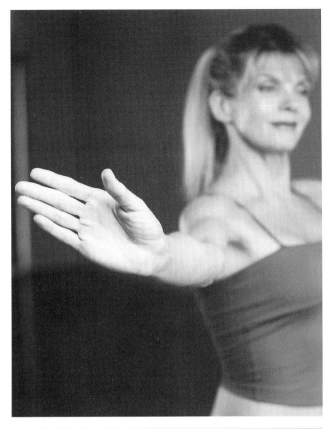
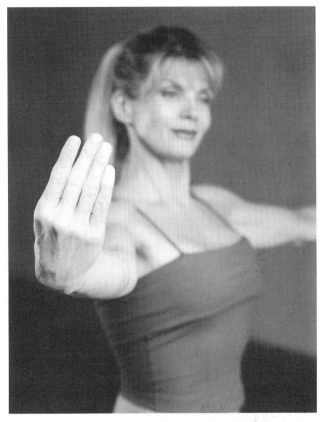
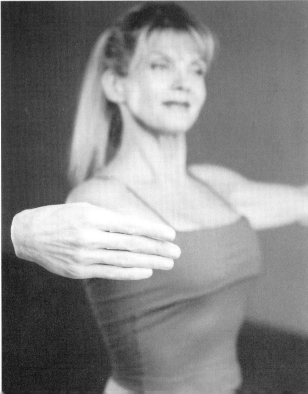
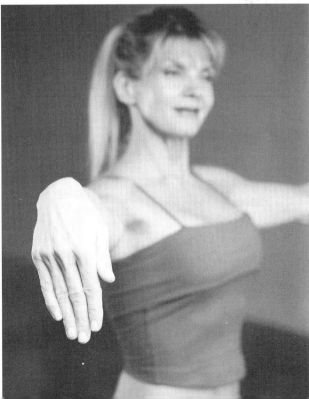

Arm Circles

MOVEMENT FOCUS: Circles in outstretched arms and shoulder joint.

REPS: Forty in each direction.

1. Begin in Mountain Pose (page 234).

2. Extend your arms out to each side, parallel to the floor.

3. Extend a line of energy through each arm, from the center of your chest out to your middle finger.

4. Circle your arms from the shoulder in four-inch circles.

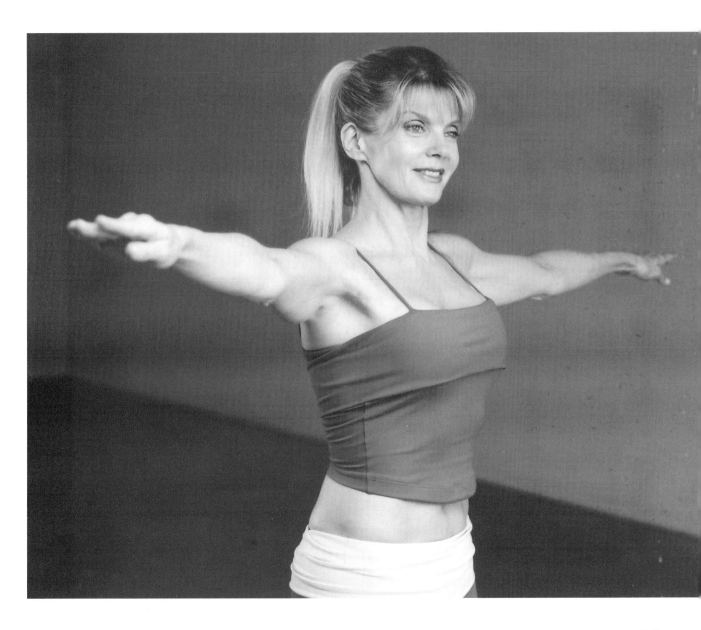

Uttanasana with Hands Interlaced Behind Back

MOVEMENT FOCUS: Stillness; legs stabilize as shoulder blades draw together.

TIME: Hold for thirty seconds.

1. Stand with your feet parallel, hip distance apart, and root your feet down into the Earth.

2. Interlace your fingers behind your back.

3. *Inhale* as you roll your shoulders down away from your ears and draw your shoulder blades toward each other.

4. *Exhale* and fold forward.

5. Pull your shoulders away from your ears as you take your arms up and over your head.

6. Keep your thighs lifted and find the release in your shoulders, back muscles, and hamstrings.

BENEFITS: Helps release and open your back body and shoulders.

NOTE: Do not lock your knees. If your hamstrings are tight or strained, bend your knees slightly.

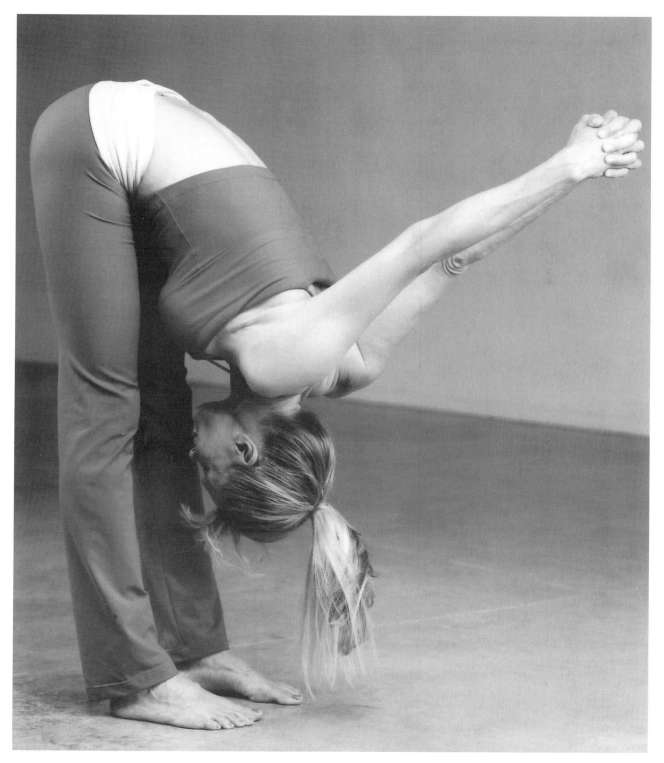

Butterfly— Wing Flap

Semicircular wave movement in upper back.

Twenty.

1. Stand with your feet hip distance apart.

2. Place your hands on top of your shoulders.

3. *Inhale* and take your elbows back, arching your upper back.

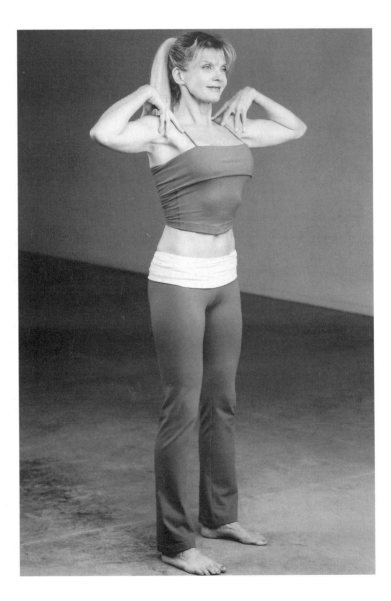

4. At the same time, move your pubic bone to your tailbone, open your chest, and lift your chin.

5. *Exhale* and draw your elbows together in front of you, while rounding your shoulders and upper back and drawing your chin to your chest.

BENEFITS: Increases range of motion in upper spine.

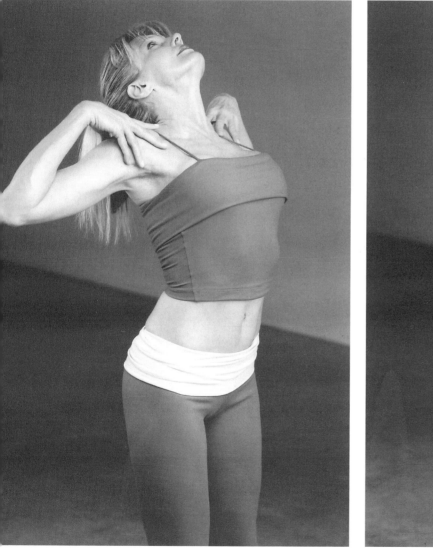 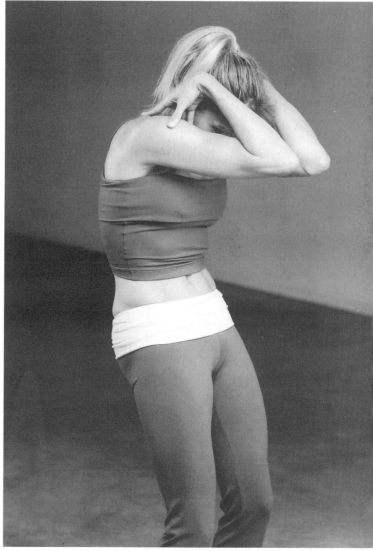

Butterfly— Elbow Circles

MOVEMENT FOCUS: Circles in upper arms and shoulder joints.

REPS: Twenty in each direction.

1. Stand with your feet hip distance apart.

2. Place your hands on top of your shoulders.

3. Trace circles with the tips of your elbows.

4. Feel into the opening of the shoulder joints.

5. Focus on creating fluid movement.

BENEFITS: Opens up a range of motion in your upper spine and shoulder joints.

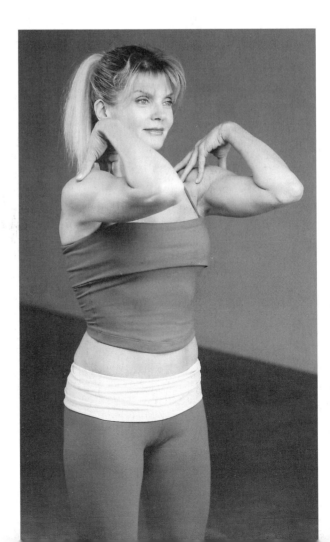

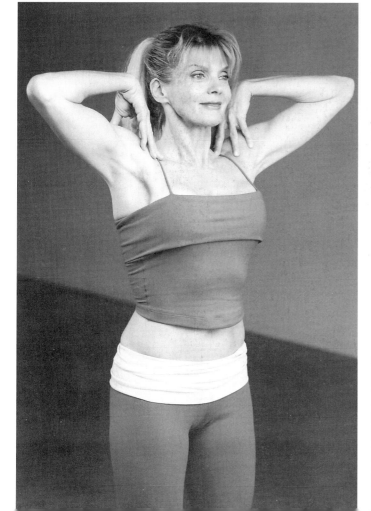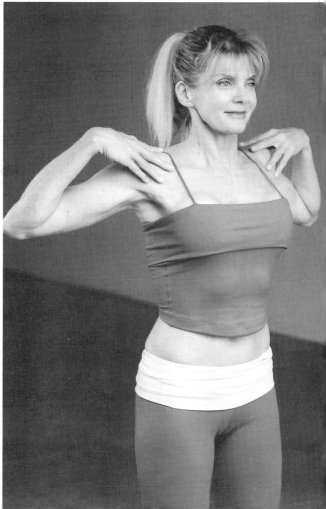

Butterfly— Twist

Upper spine twisting.

Twenty in each direction.

1. Stand with your feet hip distance apart.

2. Root your feet down into the Earth to stabilize your pelvis.

3. Place your hands on top of your shoulders.

4. Keep your elbows at shoulder height and twist your torso from side to side.

5. *Exhale,* twisting in one direction with the breath.

6. *Inhale,* coming back to the center.

7. *Exhale,* twisting to the other side with the breath.

NOTE: Twist side to side at medium speed and with attention to respecting your own spine's level of flexibility.

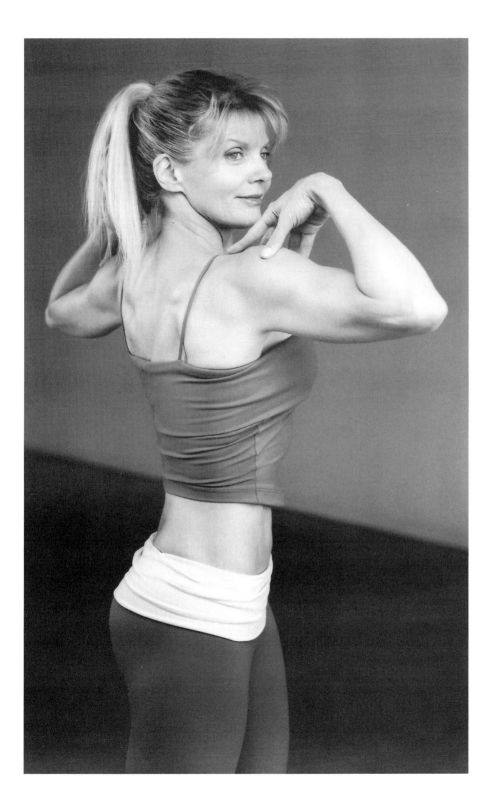

Plank

Extend spine on *inhale*; stabilize core on *exhale*.

Thirty seconds.

1. Kneel; place your wrists directly underneath your shoulders and spread your fingers.

2. Keep your shoulders over your hands as you walk your feet back, heels up and hip distance apart.

3. Press back from your navel to your heels as you draw the crown of your head forward—away from your navel.

4. Just as in Mountain Pose (page 234), the tailbone draws into the body as the thighs draw up. The lower belly lifts to support the lower back.

5. Keep your breath steady and smooth.

BEGINNING MODIFICATION: Place your knees on the floor.

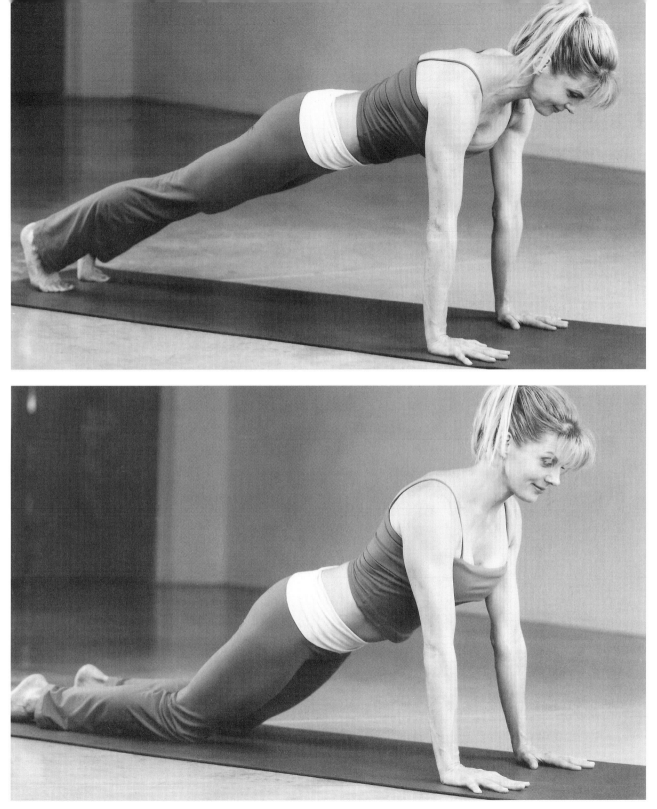

Downward Facing Dog

MOVEMENT FOCUS: Extend spine on *inhale;* stabilize core on *exhale.*

TIME: Thirty seconds.

1. Begin in Plank (page 250).

2. Press back, lift your hips, and create a right angle with your body.

3. Elongate your spine as you press back with your hands and plant your feet into the floor.

4. Focus on evenly distributing your weight between your hands and feet.

5. Press down into the heels of your palms, your thumbs, and your forefingers while stretching your fingers forward.

6. Press the heels of your feet down and stretch your toes forward.

BEGINNING MODIFICATION: Begin in a kneeling position, with your wrists under your shoulders and your knees underneath your hips, and push up into the pose.

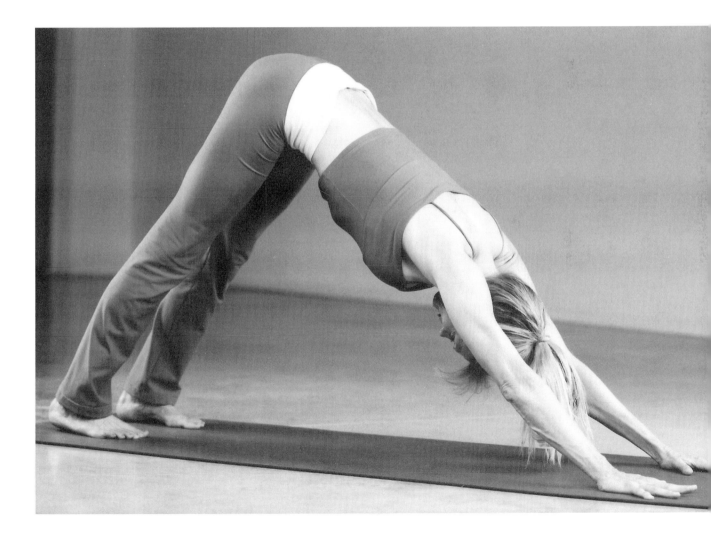

Feline Vinyasa— Moving Meditation

Vinyasa; moving with the breath.

Three cycles.

1. Come onto your hands and knees, wrists under your shoulders, knees hip distance apart underneath your hips.

2. *Exhale* as you bend your elbows toward your rib cage and lower your chest and chin to the floor.

3. *Inhale* as you pull yourself forward into Cobra (page 136), elongating your spine on the floor and lifting your chest away from the floor.

4. Draw your shoulder blades toward each other. Keep your shoulders away from your ears.

5. *Exhale,* press back onto your hands and knees, and continue to Downward Facing Dog (page 252).

6. Repeat three times.

ADVANCED MODIFICATION:

1. At step 3, pull yourself into Upward Facing Dog (photo page 257), standing on your hands and feet, shoulder distance apart, pressing down through your entire palm.

2. Roll your shoulders back.

3. Draw the bottom tips of your shoulder blades toward each other, opening your chest.

4. Lift your neck out of your shoulders as you stretch back through each leg, lifting your thighs off the floor.

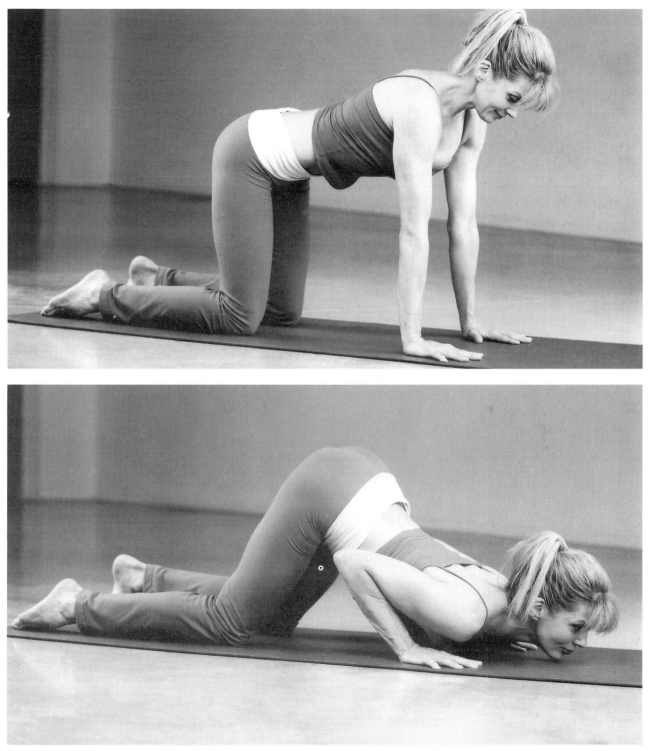

continued on next page

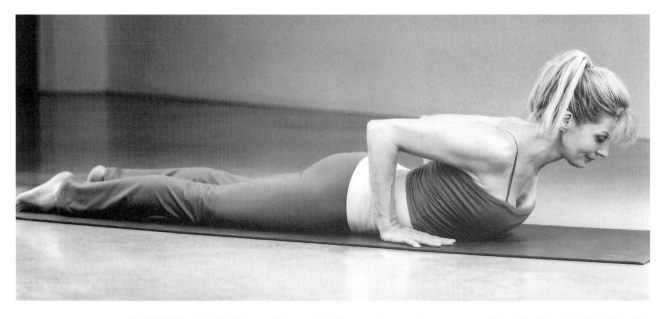

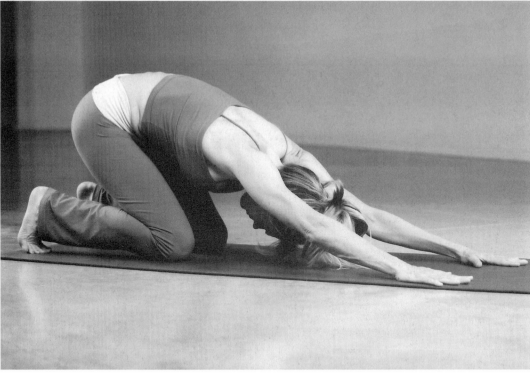

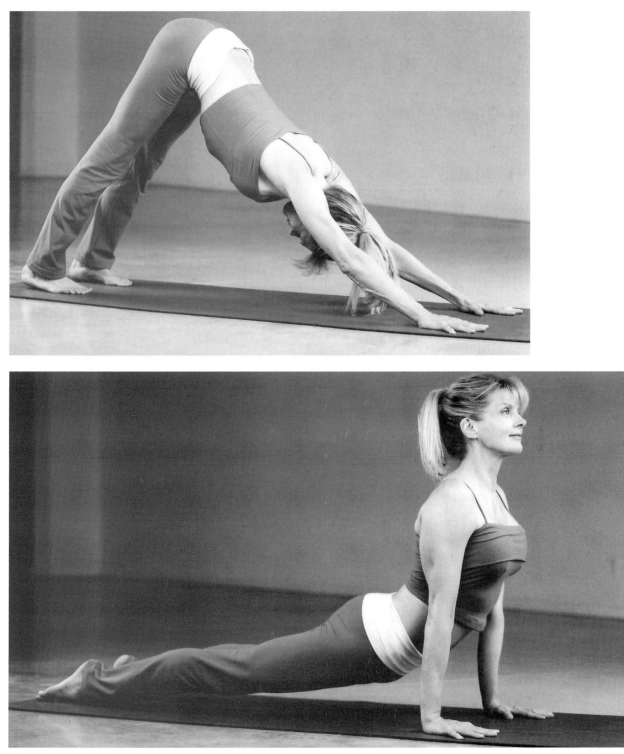

Plank Push-Ups

Internal spine elongation.

REPS: Ten, extending your spine on the *inhale,* stabilizing your core on the *exhale.*

1. Start in Plank (page 250).

2. *Inhale,* looking forward, with your lower belly lifting and your sitbones reaching toward your heels.

3. *Exhale* and bend your elbows, lowering your body until your upper arms come parallel to the floor. Keep your elbows close to your body, in line with your shoulders.

4. Keeping your core and spine stable, *inhale* and straighten your arms again into Plank.

BEGINNING MODIFICATION: Perform the same motion with your knees on the floor.

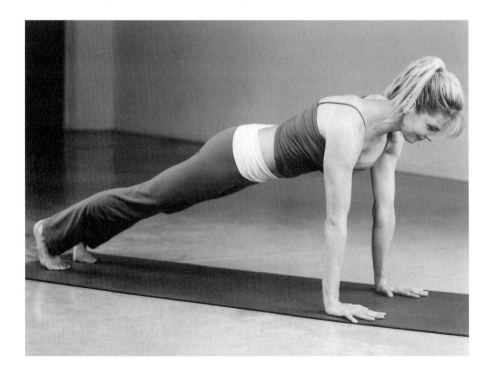

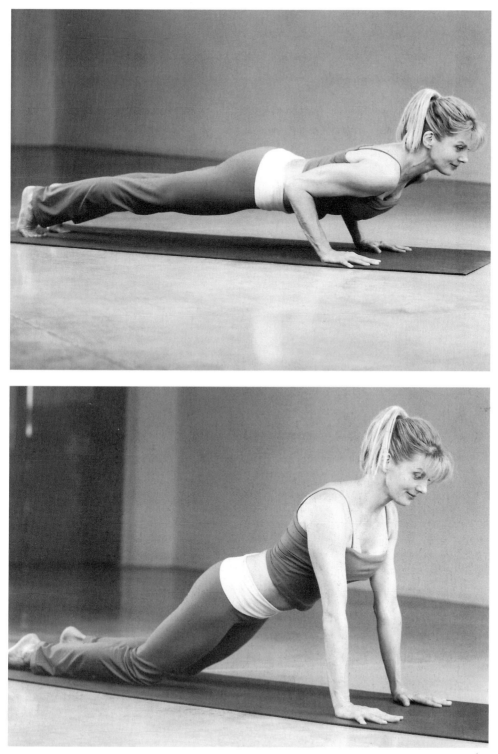

Beginning Modification

Table Pose

MOVEMENT FOCUS: Stillness; back body moving into front body.

TIME: Thirty seconds.

1. Start from a sitting position.

2. Place your feet an inch and a half in front of your sitbones.

3. Place your palms five or six inches behind your sitbones, shoulder distance apart, with your fingertips pointing toward your feet.

4. *Exhale* and lift your pelvis, bringing your whole spine parallel to the floor; draw your tailbone into your body as your inner thighs roll down toward the floor.

5. Make the front of your body flat like a table.

ADVANCED MODIFICATION (eight reps): From Table Pose, *exhale* as you curl your pubic bone toward your navel and swing your hips through your inner arms, keeping your sitbones lifted away from the floor. Repeat eight times.

BEGINNING MODIFICATION (low wrist strain): Make a fist and press down through the flat area between your first and second knuckles.

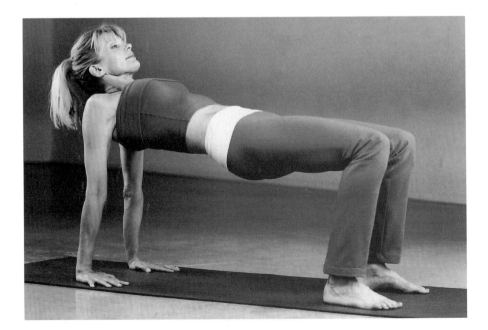

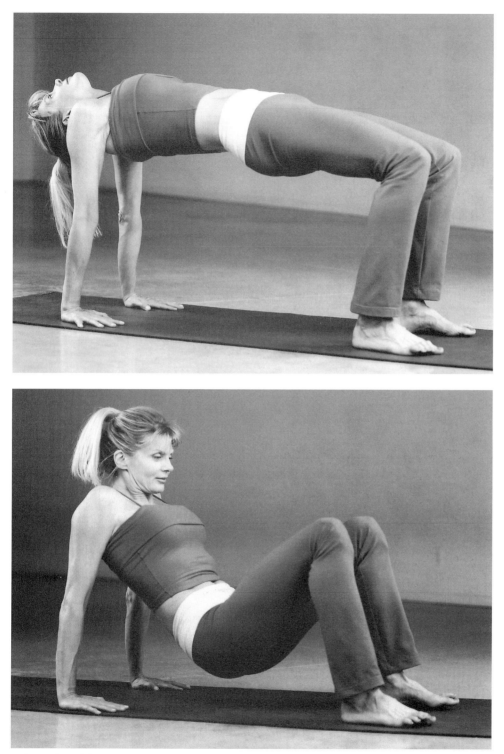

Advanced Modification

continued on next page

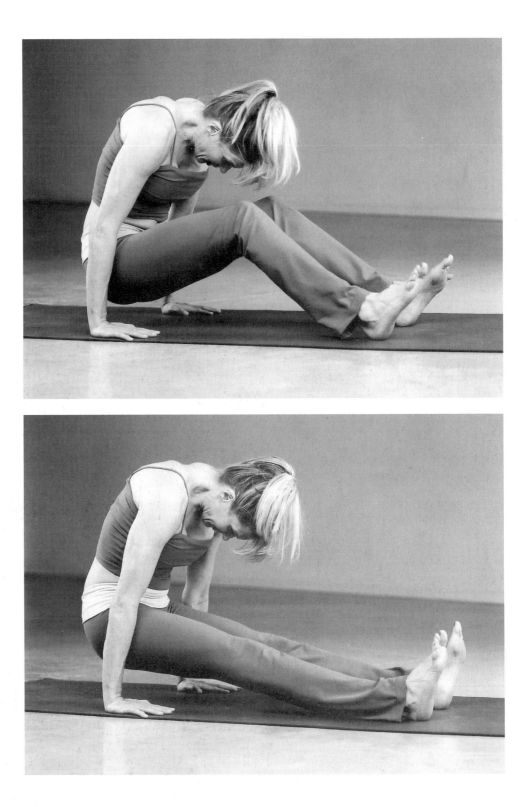

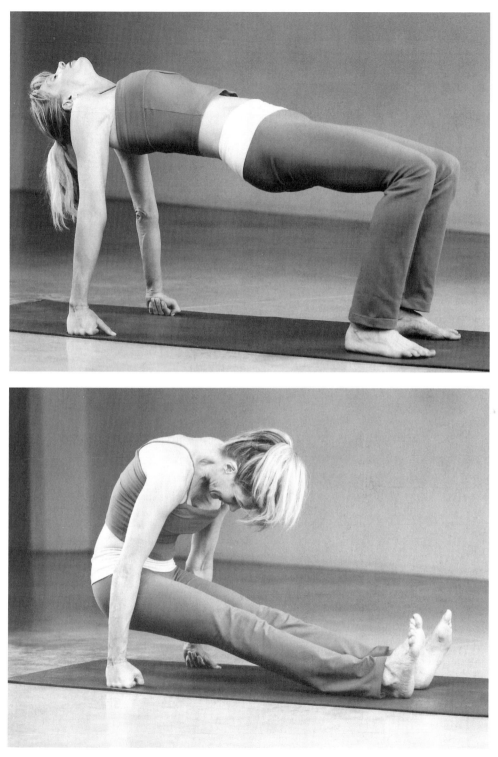

Power Cat— Pendulum

Pendulum movement of entire shoulder girdle.

Ten semicircles in each direction.

1. Start on your hands and knees with your hands a little wider than shoulder distance apart.

2. Begin to swing your shoulder girdle side to side like a pendulum, dipping your chest toward the floor as you bend your elbows.

3. Keep your movement fluid and smooth.

4. *Breathe deeply,* feeling the power of the fluid movement in your upper body and shoulders.

5. Keep your face, jaw, and neck relaxed.

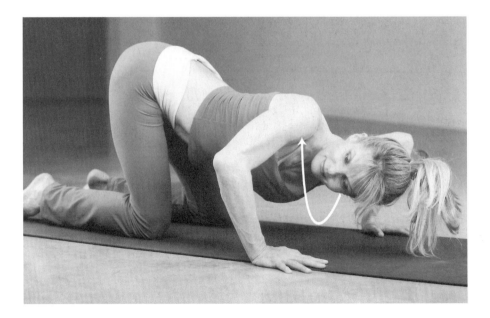

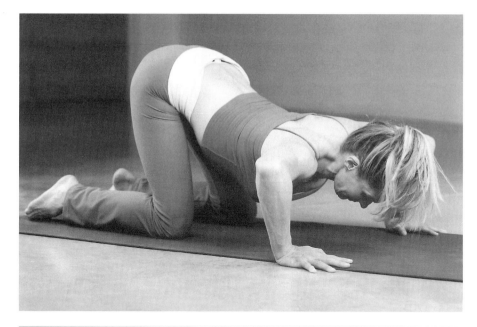

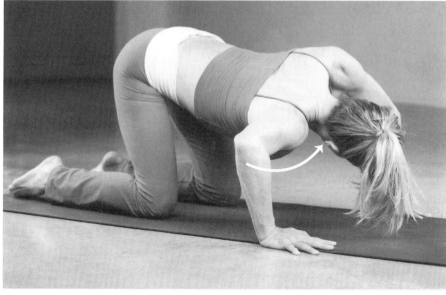

Power Cat— Circles

MOVEMENT FOCUS: Circular movement of entire shoulder girdle.

REPS: Ten circles in each direction, *inhaling* through your nose, *exhaling* through your mouth.

1. Start as in Power Cat—Pendulum (page 264).

2. Make a complete vertical circle with your shoulder girdle.

3. Notice the heat building as your entire upper torso awakens.

4. Use your breath to drive the movement.

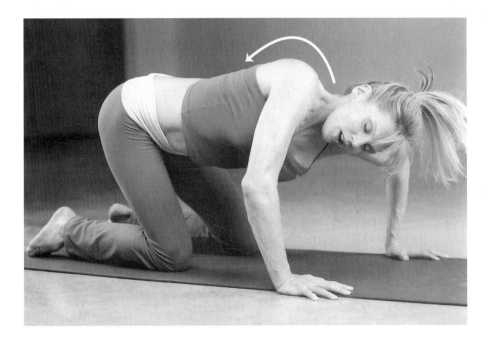

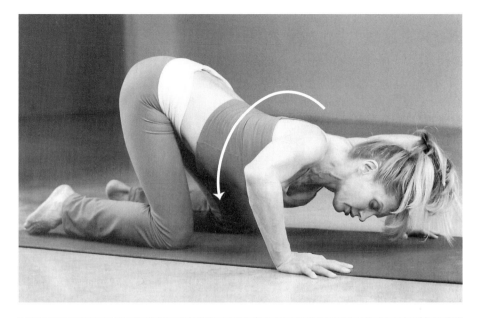

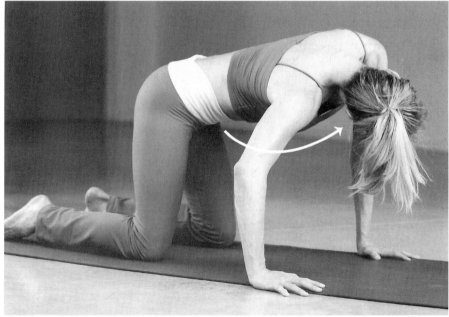

Child's Pose 2

MOVEMENT FOCUS: Stillness; yielding to Earth.

TIME: One minute.

1. Come onto your knees and shins, bringing your knees together.

2. Sit back, drawing your sitbones toward your heels.

3. Lay your chest down over your thighs and place your forehead on the floor.

4. Gently stretch your arms forward, shoulder distance apart.

5. Rest without strain. (Place a folded towel under your forehead if your head does not come to the floor.)

NOTE: If you have any knee pain, place a bed pillow behind your knees to support them.

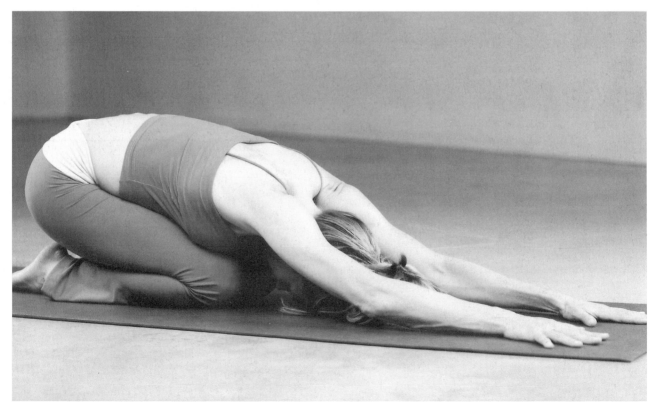

MOVEMENT FOCUS: Fluid circular movement of wrist.

REPS: Ten circles in each direction.

1. Bend your elbows in a loose, relaxed manner.

2. Make fluid circles with each wrist.

3. Let the movement ripple through each finger and into the arms.

ADVANCED MODIFICATION: As you work your upper body, feel free to add the Standing Dances that you've already learned, such as Hip Circles (page 222) or Figure-8 (page 224) in chapter 9.

Hand Dance 1— Wrist Dance

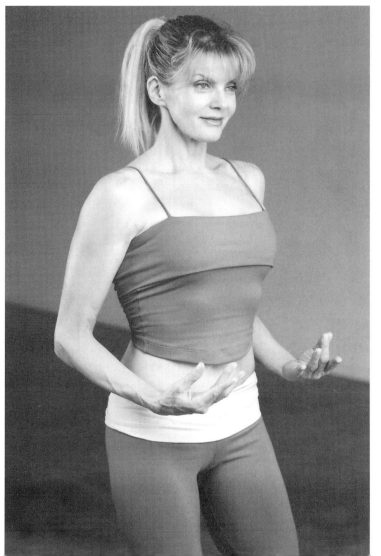

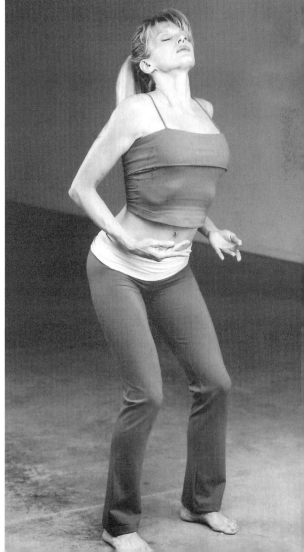

Advanced Modification

Hand Dance 2— Flamenco Wrist Dance

Fluid figure-8 movement in wrists.

Ten in each direction.

1. Lift your arms overhead in a loose, relaxed manner.

2. Make fluid figure-8s with each wrist.

3. Let the movement ripple through each finger and into your arms.

COMMENTS: As you work your upper body, feel free to add the Standing Dances that you've already learned, such as Hip Circles (page 222) or Figure-8 (page 224) in chapter 9.

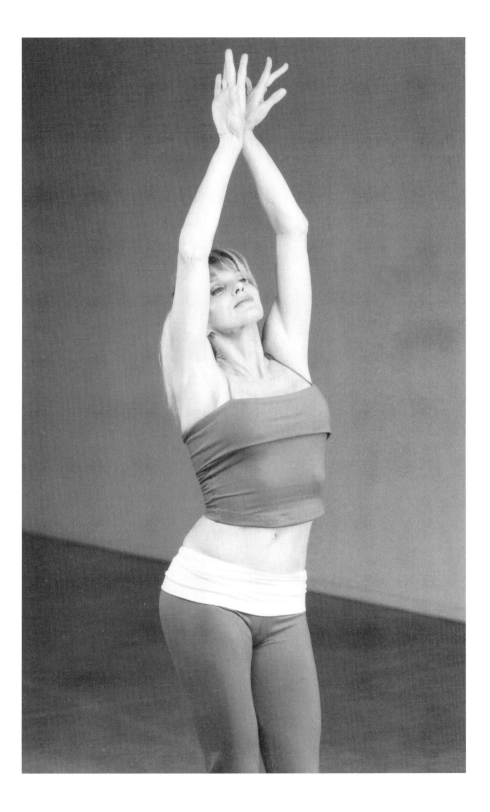

Shoulder Dance— Rolls

MOVEMENT FOCUS: Circular movement of each shoulder.

REPS: Ten in each direction, *inhaling* through your nose, *exhaling* through your mouth.

1. Make complete circles with both shoulders simultaneously.

2. Enjoy the sensation of your shoulders opening and moving in a fluid, sensual way.

COMMENTS: As you work your upper body, feel free to add the Standing Dances that you've already learned, such as Hip Circles (page 222) or Figure-8 (page 224) in chapter 9.

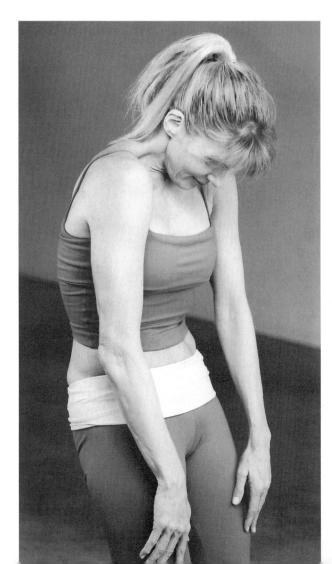
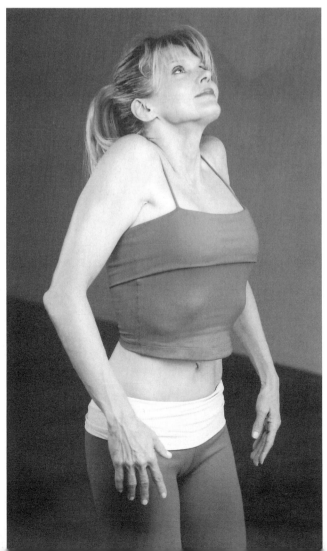

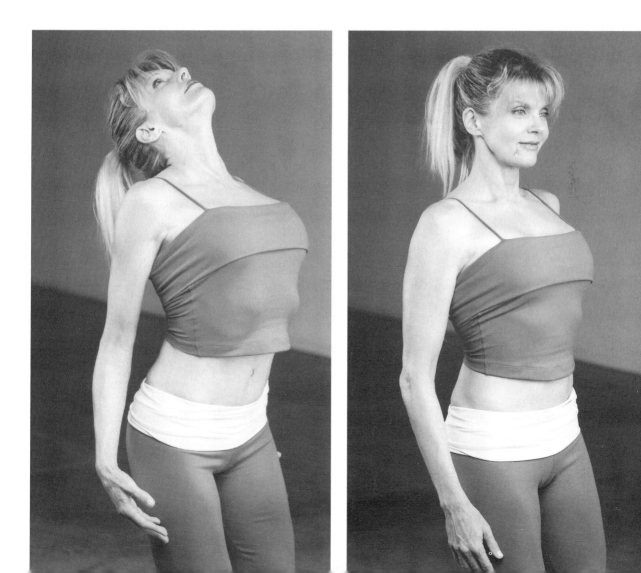

Arm Dance 1— Wings

MOVEMENT FOCUS: Semicircular movement of each arm.

REPS: Ten up and down.

1. *Imagine your arms are wings.*

2. *Inhale* as you lift both arms, leading slightly from the elbows, until your arms come shoulder distance apart overhead.

3. *Exhale* as you lower your arms, elbows dipping slightly, until your hands come to your hips.

COMMENTS: As you work your upper body, feel free to add the Standing Dances that you've already learned, such as Hip Circles (page 222) or Figure-8 (page 224) in chapter 9.

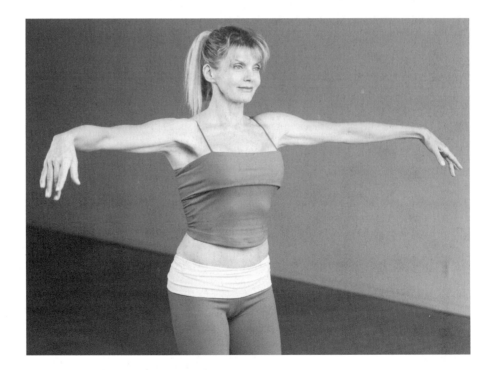

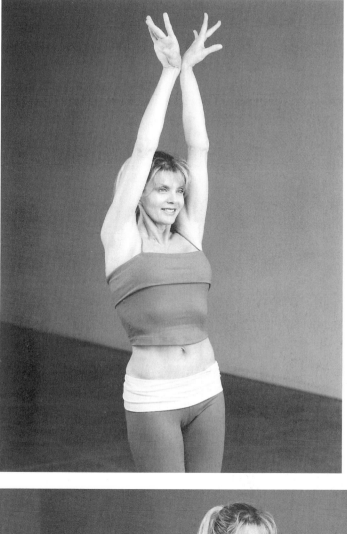

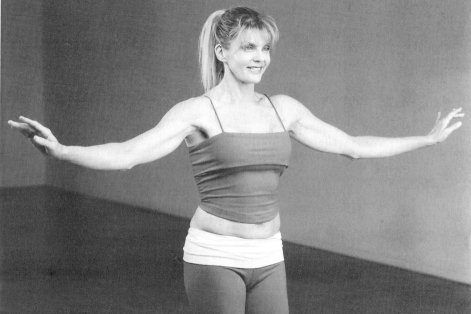

Arm Dance 2— Waves

MOVEMENT FOCUS: Alternating semicircular movement of arms.

REPS: Ten up and down on each side.

1. Begin as in Wings (page 274).

2. Alternate your arms—as one arm lifts, the other descends.

3. Focus on fluid, smooth movement.

4. Keep your shoulders and face relaxed.

COMMENTS: As you work your upper body, feel free to add the Standing Dances that you've already learned, such as Hip Circles (page 222) or Figure-8 (page 224) in chapter 9.

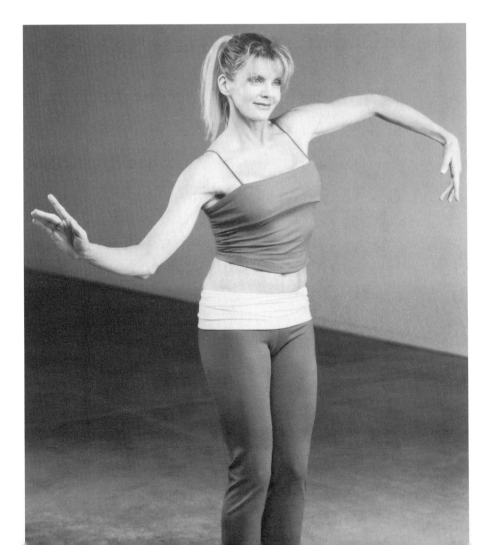

MOVEMENT FOCUS: Stillness; twisting action in spine; chest opening.

TIME: Thirty seconds on each side.

1. Stand sideways to a wall with your left foot eight inches away from the wall.

2. Step your right foot back about three or four feet.

3. Slide your left hand up the wall to a point even with your left shoulder. Keep your arm straight.

4. Keeping your shoulders down away from your ears, twist the center of your chest away from the wall.

5. Feel the release of the front of the shoulder.

6. Hold for thirty seconds and then switch sides.

Shoulder Wall Release

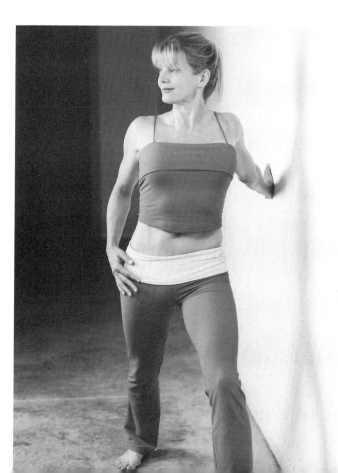

Seated Neck Release

MOVEMENT FOCUS: Stillness.

TIME: Thirty seconds on each side.

1. Sit against a wall.

2. Place your left hand, palm down, on the floor just underneath your left sitbone, fingers pointed toward the centerline of your body.

3. Press down through your entire left palm, keeping the left arm straight.

4. Keep your spine long, leaning back into the wall.

5. Reach your right hand over your head and take hold of your left ear or chin.

6. Allow the weight of your arm to draw your head toward your right shoulder.

7. As you keep your left palm pressing into the floor, feel the release on the left side of your neck.

8. Hold for thirty seconds and then switch sides.

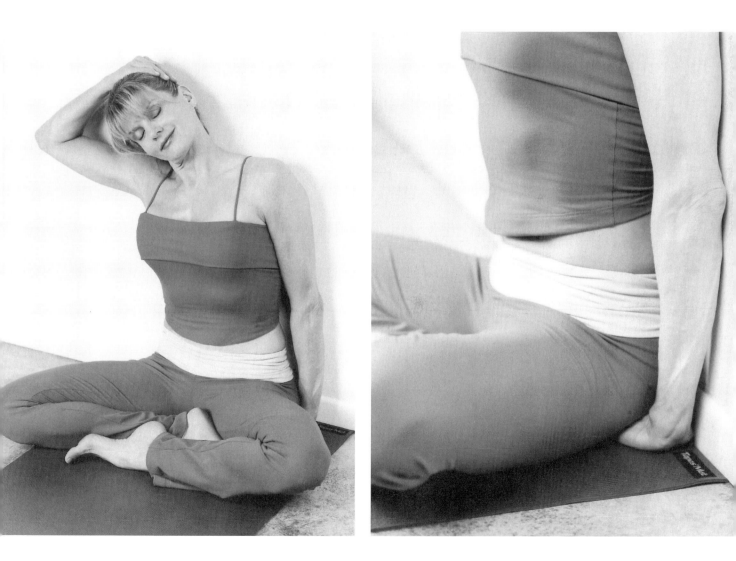

Seated Wrist Wrap

Stillness.

Thirty seconds on each side.

1. With your palms facing down, cross your right wrist over the left, then reach your palms together and interlace your fingers.

2. Pull your interlaced hands toward your body, letting your hands swing up between your arms until your knuckles point to the front again.

3. Feel the stretch along your forearms.

4. Hold for thirty seconds, then switch sides and repeat.

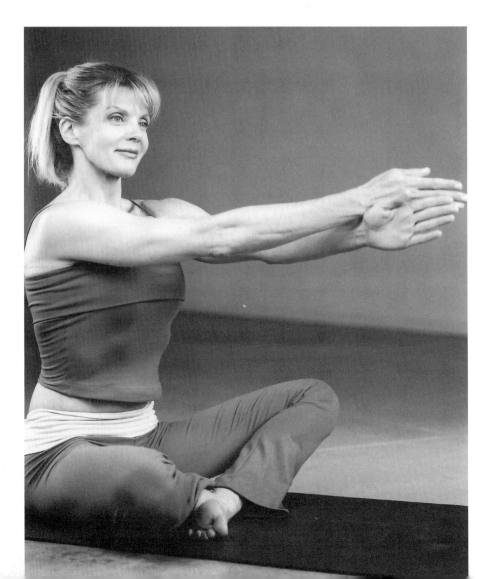

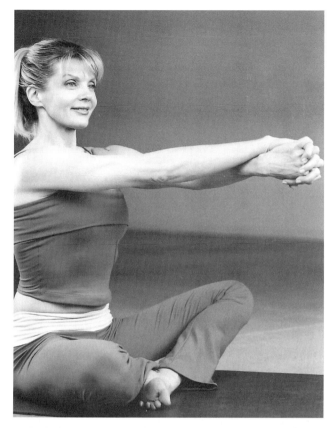

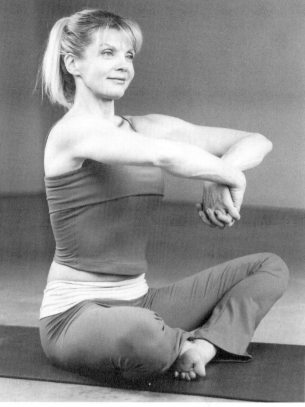

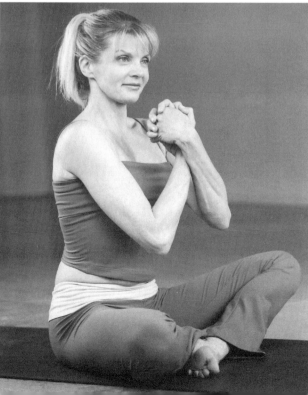

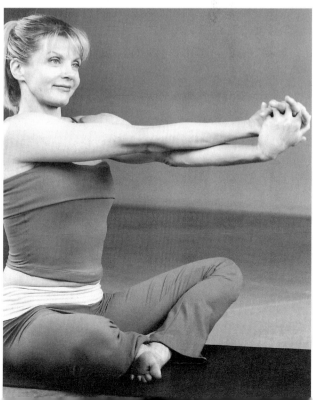

Seated Arm Wrap

MOVEMENT FOCUS: Stillness.

TIME: Thirty seconds on each side.

1. Draw your right elbow into your left elbow.

2. The right forearm stays straight; the left forearm wraps around the straight right forearm.

3. Lift your elbows from your chest and away from the floor as you roll down your back.

4. Breathe into the sensation and release between your shoulder blades.

5. Hold for thirty seconds, then switch sides and repeat.

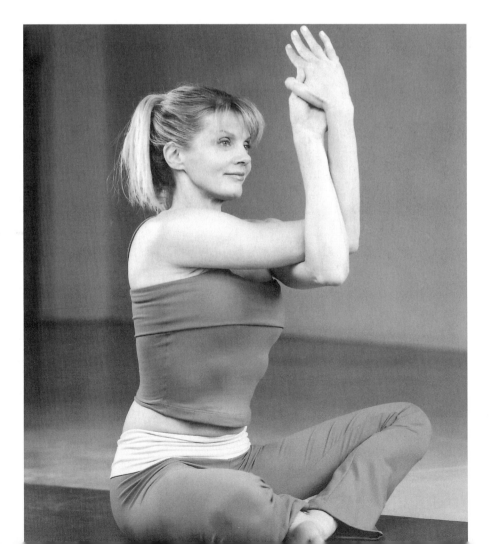

MOVEMENT FOCUS: Stillness; internal expansion of chest.

TIME: Thirty seconds on each side.

1. Sit in a comfortable cross-legged position.

2. Place your hands behind you, palms facing down.

3. Lift your back body into your front body and open up your chest, drawing your shoulder blades toward each other.

4. Keep your chin over your chest, or, if you wish, let your head tip back completely.

5. Take several deep breaths right into your chest.

Seated Heart Opener

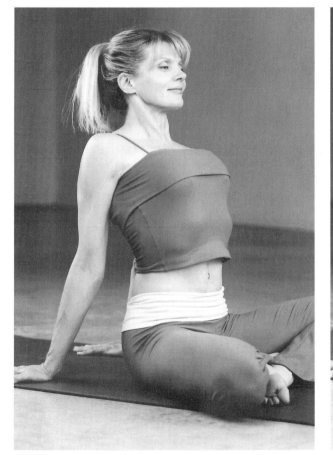

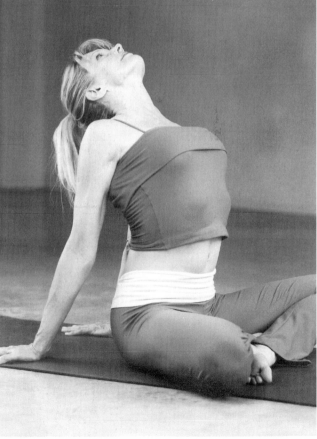

Seated Meditation

TIME: Three to five minutes.

1. Sit in a comfortable cross-legged position.

2. Place one hand on each knee or your palms together on your lap.

3. Close your eyes and go inside.

4. Relax your face, jaw, shoulders, and belly.

5. Focus on the rise and fall of your breath.

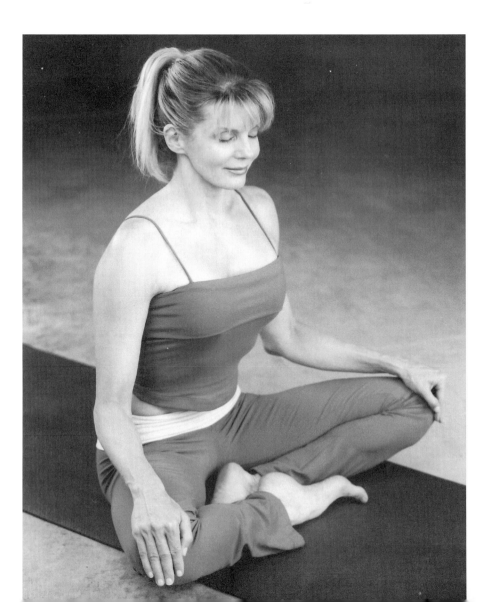

CHAPTER 11

Face and Head

Y OUR HEAD AND FACE are some of the most neglected areas of the body when it comes to releasing hidden tension and anxiety. The muscles of the jaw and face are especially prone to storing tension and can provide a quick means of releasing it with the right exercises. I love to do these exercises before public speaking events—they take only a minute, but they seem to make my whole body feel more at ease.

Lion
Breath

MOVEMENT FOCUS: Extend tongue outward toward chin.

REPS: Five, *inhaling* through your nose, *exhaling* through your mouth.

1. With your face relaxed, *inhale* deeply through your nose.

2. Stick your tongue out as far as you can toward your chin and *exhale* strongly through your mouth. Let yourself make a guttural sound as you exhale.

3. Relax your eyes and face, closing your mouth, and *inhale* deeply through your nose.

4. Repeat five times.

BENEFITS: Releases tension in the face, jaw, and throat.

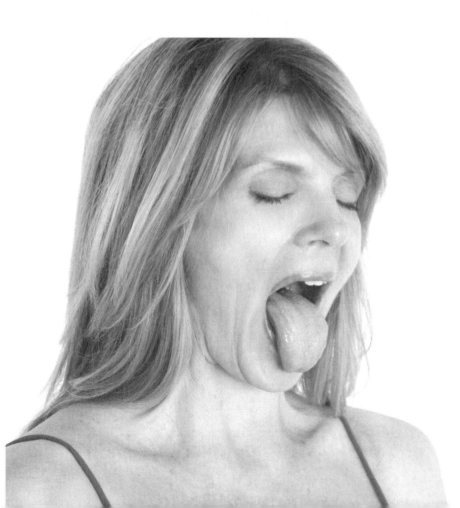

MOVEMENT FOCUS: Flutter of lips.

REPS: Five, *inhaling* through your nose, *exhaling* through your mouth with your lips together.

1. Lightly press your lips together and *inhale* through your nose.

2. Slowly *exhale* through your mouth, causing your lips to flutter like a horse.

3. Feel the skin around your mouth and cheeks fluttering and releasing as well.

BENEFITS: Releases tension in the face and lips.

Horse
Breath

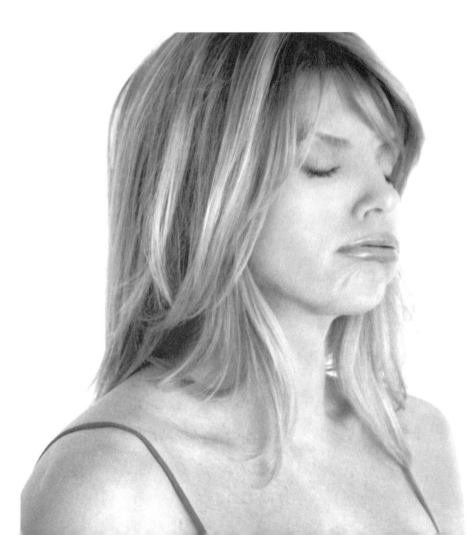

Jaw Release

Gentle stretching of the jaw muscles.

Five in each direction.

1. Jut your lower jaw forward.

2. Draw your jaw all the way to the right, and then to the left.

3. Keep the movement smooth and your jaw relaxed.

Releases jaw muscles; helps relax TMJ (temporomandibular joint).

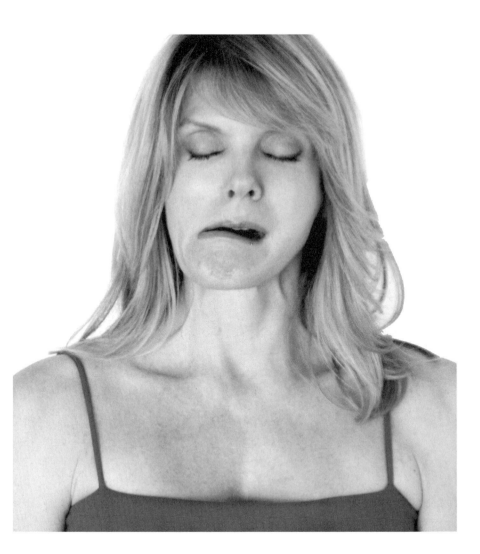

MOVEMENT FOCUS: Gentle stretching of neck muscles.

REPS: Ten to thirty seconds on each side.

1. Standing or seated upright, tilt your right ear to your right shoulder and draw your right arm up around your head. Allow the weight of the arm to gently stretch your neck and create a release.

2. Breathe smoothly and steadily.

3. If you find an area that feels tight, stuck, or painful, slow down and draw your awareness to that area. What do you feel there? What is the texture of the sensation? Saturate the area with your entire awareness and feel into it.

BENEFITS: Releases tension in the muscles around your throat, neck, and upper back.

Neck Release

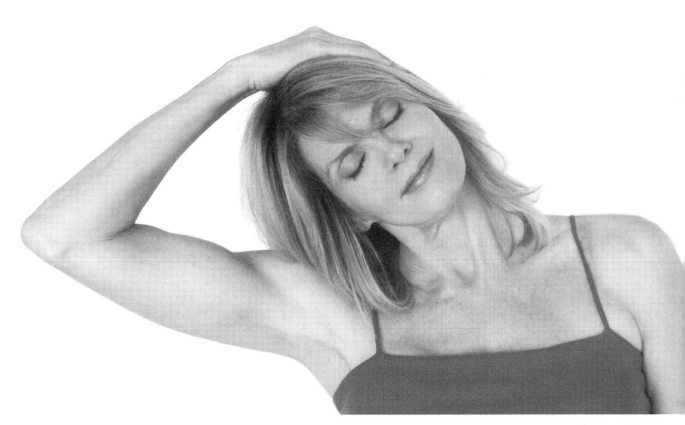

Eye Rolls

Circles with eyes.

Five circles in each direction.

1. Keeping your head still, make the widest possible circles with your eyes.

Releases tension in the eyes, relaxes eye muscles.

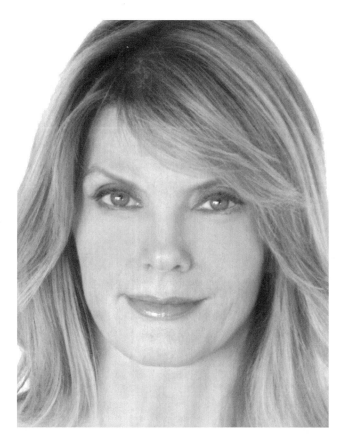

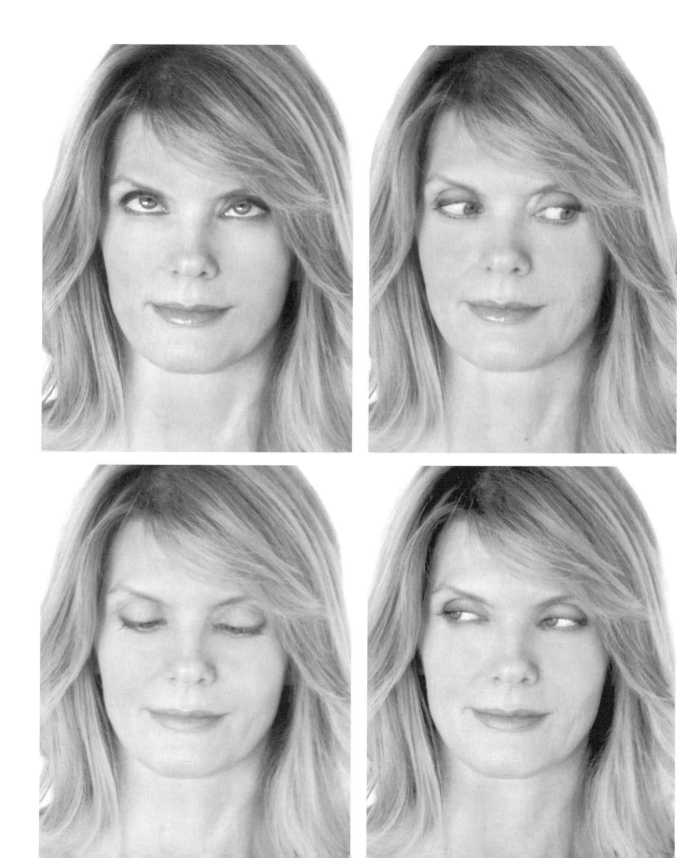

Facial Massage

MOVEMENT FOCUS: Circular massage patterns with fingers on skull, face, and jaw.

TIME: Three minutes.

1. Interlace your fingers over the top of your head so that your thumbs come to your temples.

2. Make circular movements at each temple.

3. Place your thumbs together at the bridge of your nose and spread them outward just underneath your brow ridge.

4. Place your thumbs together at the bridge of your nose and draw them straight up your forehead toward your hairline and outward toward your temples.

5. Spreading your fingers on your skull, massage your jawline, especially the large muscles where your upper and lower jaws meet.

6. Massage your skull, making small circles with each finger.

BENEFITS: Total relaxation.

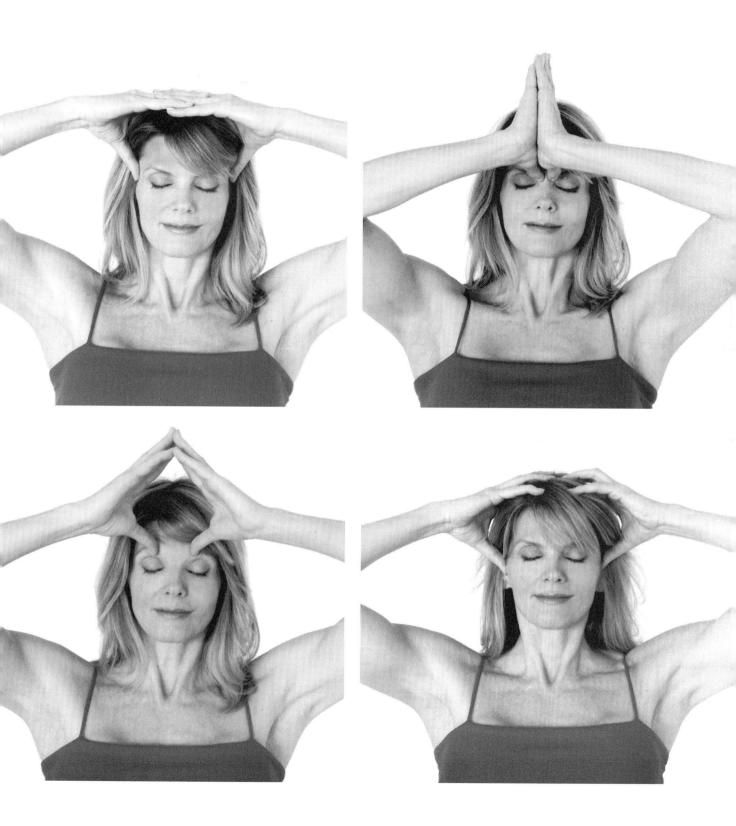

Viparita Karani

MOVEMENT FOCUS: Stillness.

TIME: Three minutes.

1. Lie down with your sitbones against a wall and your legs extended, feet together.

2. Your lower back should be flat on the floor. If necessary, start with your sitbones slightly away from the wall in order to keep your lower back flat.

3. Place your palms on your belly and breathe deeply.

4. Expand your chest as you feel into the opening of your abdomen and chest.

5. Rest completely as you let the wall support you.

BENEFITS: Restores the body without muscular effort.

BEGINNING MODIFICATION: Lie down, resting your legs with bent knees over a chair or a bed.

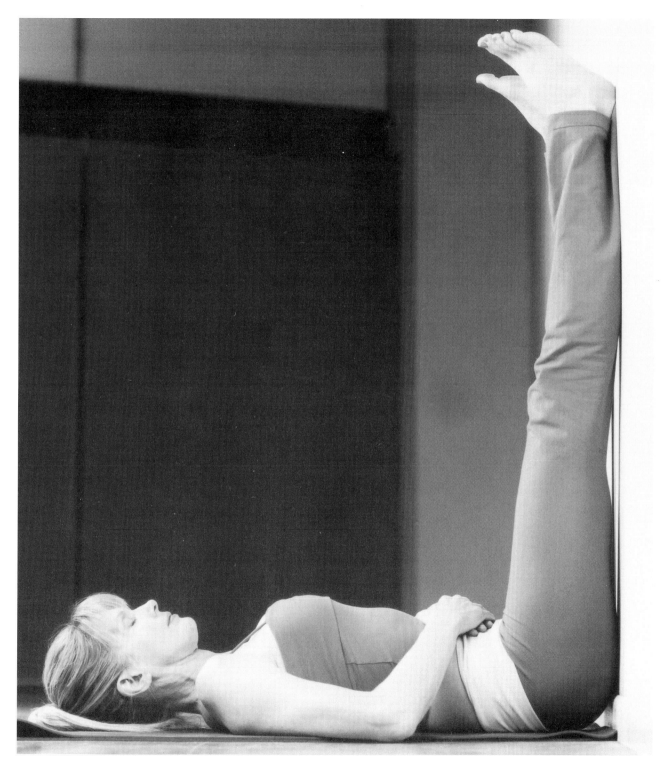

Savasana Full-Body Meditation

Stillness.

Three to five minutes.

1. Lie down on your back.

2. Relax your shoulders away from your ears and allow the weight of your bones to surrender to the support of the Earth.

3. Allow a wave of relaxation to wash over you from the top of your head all the way to your toes.

4. Breathe softly and slowly.

5. Soften and relax your facial muscles, eyes, lips, tongue, and jaw.

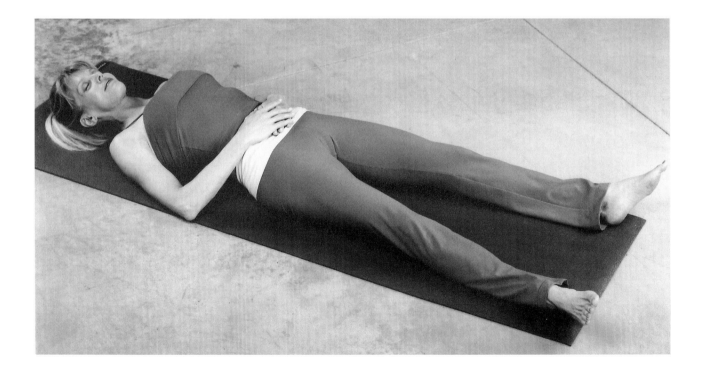

CHAPTER 12

Special Routines

Special Routine 1: Fluid Relaxation Meditation

Special Routine 2: Sensual Strength and Weight Loss

Opening Floor Flow

Sensual Strength Flow

Closing Release Flow

Special Routine 3: *Flex Appeal* Dance

Opening

Floor Dance Work

Standing Dance Work

Resources and Recommended Reading

Books

Alive and Well: A Workbook for Recovering Your Body; Rita Justice, Ph.D.; Peak Press, 1996

Aphrodite's Daughters: Women's Sexual Stories and the Journey of the Soul; Jalaja Bonheim; Fireside, 1997

Awareness Through Movement: Easy-to-Do Health Exercises to Improve Your Posture, Vision, Imagination, and Personal Awareness; Moshe Feldenkrais; HarperCollins, 1990

Bioenergetics: The Revolutionary Therapy That Uses the Language of the Body to Heal the Problems of the Mind; Alexander Lowen, M.D.; Penguin Books, 1975

Bodymind; Ken Dychtwald; Jeremy P. Tarcher Inc., 1986

Flow — The Psychology of Optimal Experience: Steps Toward Enhancing the Quality of Life; Mihaly Csikszentmihalyi; HarperPerennial, 1990

Luna Yoga: Vital Fertility and Sexuality; Adelheid Ohlig; Ash Tree Publishing, 1994

Moving Toward Life: Five Decades of Transformational Dance; Anna Halprin; University Press of New England, 1995

Sacred Woman, Sacred Dance: Awakening Spirituality Through Movement and Ritual; Iris J. Stewart; Inner Traditions, 2000

Self-Esteem: A Proven Program of Cognitive Techniques for Assessing, Improving, and Maintaining Your Self-Esteem; Matthew McKay, Ph.D., and Patrick Fanning; New Harbinger Publications, 2000

When the Drummers Were Women: A Spiritual History of Rhythm; Layne Redmond; Three Rivers Press, 1997

Women Who Run with the Wolves: Myths and Stories of the Wild Woman Archetype; Clarissa Pinkola Estés, Ph.D.; Ballantine Books, 1992

Music

www.zendancing.com for hot world music to inspire your *Flex Appeal* workout

Index

About the Authors

Kathy Smith has been a visionary in the fitness industry for more than twenty years. She is among the top sellers of fitness videos, audiotapes, books, and equipment and contributes to *Self* magazine, supporting her mission of educating consumers on being healthy and fit. Smith's more than thirty award-winning videos have sold more than twelve million copies around the world, earning her a place in the Video Hall of Fame. She has been at the forefront of promoting sports and fitness to America's youth and serves on the board of directors of the highly acclaimed University Elementary School at the University of California, Los Angeles. She is also a national ambassador for the March of Dimes. Smith is currently a member of the Woman's Sports Foundation's board of stewards, and she served on the board of trustees from 1993 to 1996. Her company, Kathy Smith Lifestyles, established a scholarship fund through the Woman's Sports Foundation in the name of her two daughters, Kate and Perrie, which demonstrates Smith's ongoing commitment to promoting sports and fitness to young girls. *Kathy Smith's Flex Appeal* is Smith's sixth book. Her previous five were *Kathy Smith's Moving Through Menopause, Kathy Smith's Lift Weights to Lose Weight, Kathy Smith's Getting Better All the Time, Kathy Smith's Fitness Makeover,* and *Kathy Smith's WalkFit for a Better Body.*

Robert Miller is a freelance writer and composer with extensive experience in the areas of health and fitness. He is the coauthor of *Kathy Smith's Lift Weights to Lose Weight* and *Kathy Smith's Moving Through Menopause,* and served as executive producer for *Kathy Smith's Lift Weights to Lose Weight 2, Kathy Smith's The Rules of Fatburning,* and *Kathy Smith's Flex Appeal.* Miller was editorial director for Health for Life Publications from 1984 through 1999 (www.infinitecanon.com).

Micheline Berry is a yoga teacher, dancer, and award-winning filmmaker and has guided more than 350 live world music/ecstatic dance events since 1996. She is the founder of Zen Dancing®, a highly recognized world music and dance event, and is one of the founding producers of Shaman's Dream World Groove Ensemble. Berry leads yoga, world music, dance, and eco-adventure retreats internationally and is based in Venice, California, where she teaches at Sacred Movement, Center for Yoga and Healing. Her work has appeared in *Harper's Bazaar, Shape Magazine,* and *Los Angeles Magazine,* and has been featured on the BBC and Lifetime Television (www.michelineberry.com or www.zendancing.com).